also by CATHERINE O'NEILL GRACE:

*Best Friends, Worst Enemies: Understanding the
Social Lives of Children*
(with Michael Thompson, Ph.D.
and Lawrence J. Cohen, Ph.D.)

*Mom, They're Teasing Me: Helping Your Child
Solve Social Problems*
(with Michael Thompson, Ph.D.
and Lawrence J. Cohen, Ph.D.)

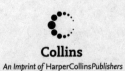

Collins
An Imprint of HarperCollinsPublishers

Why Is My Baby Crying?

Why Is My Baby Crying?

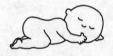

THE PARENT'S SURVIVAL GUIDE FOR
COPING WITH CRYING PROBLEMS AND COLIC

Barry M. Lester, Ph.D.

WITH CATHERINE O'NEILL GRACE

WHY IS MY BABY CRYING? Copyright © 2005 by Barry M. Lester, Ph.D. All rights reserved. Printed in the United States of America. No part of this book may be used or reproduced in any manner whatsoever without written permission except in the case of brief quotations embodied in critical articles and reviews. For information, address HarperCollins Publishers, 10 East 53rd Street, New York, NY 10022.

HarperCollins books may be purchased for educational, business, or sales promotional use. For information, please write: Special Markets Department, HarperCollins Publishers, 10 East 53rd Street, New York, NY 10022.

First Collins paperback edition published 2006

Designed by Gretchen Achilles

The Library of Congress has catalogued the hardcover edition as follows:

Lester, Barry M.
    Why is my baby crying? : the parent's survival guide for coping with crying problems and colic / Barry M. Lester with Catherine O'Neill Grace.
        p.   cm.
    ISBN 0-06-052714-5
    1. Colic.   2. Crying in infants.   3. Infants (Newborn)—Care.
I. Grace, Catherine O'Neill, 1950–   II. Title.
RJ267.L47   2005
618.92'09755—dc22

                                                    2004047597

ISBN-10: 0-06-055671-4
ISBN-13: 978-0-06-055671-6

06 07 08 09 10   WBC/RRD   10 9 8 7 6 5 4 3 2 1

To my wife, LYN, and the kids,

NATANIEL, ANDRES, and GABBY—the best people on the planet

ACKNOWLEDGMENTS

I have been carrying some version of this book around in my head for almost 30 years. It all began in 1971 in Guatemala, where I spent several years studying malnourished babies and was haunted by their crying. I have been conducting research about infant crying ever since. I have studied the cries of all kinds of populations, including babies with medical conditions such as prematurity or drug exposure, babies who later died of sudden infant death syndrome, normal babies, and babies with colic. During these decades, I have worked with an engineering group to develop the only computer analysis system for the acoustical interpretation of infant cries. I have studied babies' parents to see how they react to and feel about their own baby's cries as well as the cries of other babies.

Throughout the years, parents kept on asking me about crying and colic. I didn't feel comfortable treating the families in the context of my research studies. But I realized that these parents were desperate, and I knew I could help. So in 1986 I set up a colic clinic at Women & Infants Hospital in Providence, Rhode Island. It remains the only clinic in the country dedicated to colic. I chaired the first-ever pediatric roundtable on colic and the first-ever roundtable on colic and crying for practitioners. But I didn't want to keep what I knew among a few professionals and myself. For me, this book was the next step. It is time to share what I know with the parents whose lives feel wrecked by their colicky babies.

Four million babies are born in the United States each year. Of these infants, some 20 percent will have the symptoms of excessive crying/colic. That could mean as many as 800,000 parents with colicky babies, 800,000 mothers who may wind up with a disturbed relationship with their baby, 800,000 fathers who may feel helpless, 800,000 couples who may have marital problems, and 800,000 mothers-in-law offering free advice. At the Colic Clinic, we see only a fraction of these families. We want to help more people. That's one reason why I wrote this book. But I also wrote it because to understand colic, you also need to understand crying and how crying and colic makes a difference in your relationship with your baby.

This is a deeply personal book that I wrote as if I were talking directly to you—parents who want to know about crying and colic. Although the words are mine, what you will read was shaped by some extraordinary people. First of all, I thank the many parents who shared their pain, their hopes, their fears about themselves and their babies, their wisdom, and even their humor. You've heard that overused phrase, "Whatever doesn't kill you, makes you stronger." Well, the fact is that the strength that families have found in coping with a colicky baby has made them better parents.

The other extraordinary people are those I have worked with over the years. Zack Boukydis and Jayne Cucca started the Colic Clinic with me in 1986 and over the years helped develop the model of providing both medical and psychological services. Pam High has strengthened the pediatric and sleep components of the program, and Jean Twomey adds depth to parenting and family issues. We have also learned from Rose Bigsby in occupational therapy and Susan Dickstein in psychology.

My years with Dr. Berry Brazelton before I came to Brown Medical School provided a foundation for the clinical approach we use here. Sandy Zeskind made me aware of the importance of the way parents perceive their babies' cries. Dave Schnarch helped me find the courage to write this book. And without Lyn's support, I would be crying because this book never would have happened. I thank you all. And thanks, Mom.

—BARRY LESTER

Providence, Rhode Island

September 2003

CONTENTS

Contents

CHAPTER ONE

No Language but a Cry: What Your Baby Is Trying to Tell You

An infant crying in the night:
An infant crying for the light:
And with no language but a cry.

—ALFRED, LORD TENNYSON

rying is normal. Colic is not. People who say that colic is normal not only are wrong; they also are doing a huge disservice to families who have colicky babies. Those families know it is anything but normal. Being told it is normal just makes those parents feel like there is something wrong with them. But it is true that to understand colic you first need to understand normal crying. So in this book, we will keep moving back and forth between crying and colic.

Within the first 5 minutes of a baby's birth, the doctor examines the newborn and assigns an Apgar score as a measure of the baby's health. The Apgar is scored on five dimensions: heart rate, respiration, muscle tone, reflex response, and skin color. A baby gets 0, 1, or 2 on each dimension, so the highest score—the "perfect" baby—is a 10. A good strong cry rates a 2 on the respiration scale. Getting a 0 means the baby is simply breathing, and this is considered a bad thing.

A good cry indicates that a large part of the baby's physiological system is intact and functioning well. Crying requires a baby to perform a complicated and sophisticated set of physiological activities that involve the brain and the respiratory, motor, and vocal systems. Crying helps physiology by increasing pulmonary (lung) capacity. The baby gets more active when he cries, which increases muscle activity, generates heat, and helps the baby regulate his temperature. (What do babies do when they're cold? They cry. This generates heat and they warm up.)

We want babies to cry. Crying means a baby is robust, is intact, has energy, and can communicate. Physicians even talk about an infant's "respiratory effort"—a strong, lusty cry. When babies don't cry or when their cry is abnormal, this can mean there is something wrong.

Little babies can't talk with words, so for them the cry is their language. We are used to thinking that communication means language, as in words and sentences, and that you have to have language to communicate. (In fact, the word *infancy* comes from the Latin *infans*, which means "speechless.") But speech, or language, has two components. The first is the words themselves and their syntax (the grammar and all that stuff we hated to learn in school but which turns out to be quite useful because, after all, we are able to communicate). The second component of language is its prosodic features: pitch, loudness, melody, and intonation. In a sense, these prosodic features carry our feelings. Cry is all prosody. Babies don't have the words, but they sure have the feelings—and they communicate their feelings, their needs, and their wants through the prosodic features of pitch, loudness, melody, and intonation. Crying is a baby's first way of communicating. It is the language the baby uses before words.

Our job as parents is to understand our babies' cry language. We need to correctly interpret it so that we can figure out what the baby wants and respond accordingly. Our job is much more complicated than the baby's is. First we have to interpret the little tyke's screams. Then we have to figure out an action plan—what he needs, how to implement it, and how to provide the right kind of parenting. The baby's job is simpler. (After all, he's only a baby.) The baby has to tell us what's on his mind, what he needs, and make sure that he is communicating well by sending out clear and unambiguous signals so we can tell from his cry what's up. The only way he can mess up (and I'm not talking diapers) is to have an unusual or even abnormal cry. Right from birth, a baby is crying to tell us about his medical or neurological state.

What is an abnormal cry? A very high-pitched cry usually signals abnormality and can mean that the baby has a neurological problem—a problem in the brain. For example, there is a syndrome called cri du chat (the term is French and means "cry of the cat"), a very rare genetic problem in which the cry is high-pitched and almost hollow-sounding. But the sound is so distinctive that the condition is virtually diagnosed from the cry. Fortunately, this is a rare chromosomal disorder. I have only seen and heard three of these babies in my career, but the sound of their cries literally sent chills down my spine.

There are a few other situations when we know that something is wrong with a baby from the cry. Sometimes, and this too is rare, babies are asphyxiated because of lack of oxygen during birth, and the brain is damaged. These infants also have very high-pitched cries.

There are important parallels between abnormal, normal, and colic cries.

Think about why an ambulance siren gets our attention. Humans are particularly responsive to higher-pitched sounds—the maximum acoustic response of the ear is above 800 Hertz (cycles per second). And sirens are not only high-pitched; they change, they are dynamic. So are baby cries. What gets us going in a baby's cry is its high-pitched, warbling sound. Sounds at certain frequencies make people sit up and take notice. This is part of the biology of the human auditory system. In fact, there are evolutionary biologists who argue that a baby's cries are programmed to be at certain pitch levels to ensure the baby's survival! When parents hear that loud, high-pitched cry, they can't help but look around to see what's wrong.

The cry is an information transmission system that sends affective messages—hunger, pain, and need for attention. Crying has been called an acoustical umbilical cord that keeps the infant close to the mother. Ethologists, scientists who study animal behavior, call crying "a proximity-promoting and maintaining signal"—that is, it encourages the mother to stay with and soothe her baby.

Crying has a very basic biological-evolutionary purpose. In the animal kingdom, there are lots of critters that can immediately walk, swim, or otherwise get around at birth, so when they need Mom, they can just boogie up to her. But relative to other species, human babies have a long period of dependency. So we depend exclusively on vocal communication to signal distress, to tell Mom when we need her, alert her when we are in trouble, and summon her when we want to be close. Crying turns out to be an exceptionally effective survival mechanism. Spiders have legs; babies have crying. Spiders walk to Mom; babies cry and Mom comes. It works!

Moreover, each cry is individual. Studies have found that mothers can pick out their baby's cry from another's. Even in the hospital, a new mom wakes only when her baby cries. In this way, infants are programmed from birth to solicit care from their parents, and their parents are programmed to know how to read their baby's cry signal and know what to do.

Many animal species—including cats, bats, elephants, seals, and reindeer, as well as humans—use a distress cry to signal the mother when the infant is isolated, hungry, or cold. One animal researcher even took some of the infant cry prints from our lab and demonstrated that they looked almost the same as the cry a kitten made when it was isolated from its mother. When the big (momma) cat hears this cry, she retrieves her baby kitten and brings it back to safety and comfort.

But there's more. Have you ever wondered how opera singers are able to project their voices so that they carry throughout a theater and can be heard without a microphone and above the orchestra? Singers use something called "singer formant," which means they shift their voice into a higher vocal register to which human hearing is more sensitive. You guessed it—it's the same vocal register as sirens and baby cries!

Crying is the language of the newborn and it is designed to get our attention. Think of what happens when this system works correctly. Baby cries. (Let's not worry about why the baby is crying at this point.) Mom (usually) comes and picks up baby. Baby stops crying. Baby gets what she wanted. And Mom gets doubly rewarded. First, the baby stopped crying. Second, it was her doing, her care, that made this happen. This reinforces her feeling of being an effective, competent mother and enhances her self-esteem.

Now let's kick it up a notch. Let's say that not only does

the baby stop crying but she also opens her eyes and looks right at Mom. Their eyes meet, not just for a fleeting glance but for a moment of intensity, of intimacy, of love. I'm not going to even give the baby the smile yet. After all, this is a newborn. The smile will come later. But just this eye contact is a bonus—and all because Mom picked up her crying baby.

We've just learned something else about crying: Crying triggers social interaction. It enables you and your baby to better know each other. From a biological-evolutionary perspective, we might even say that part of the attention-getting aspect of the cry is to facilitate social interaction. Babies are programmed to cry not only to have their physical needs taken care of but to have their emotional needs attended to as well.

What a great system. What starts out as a negative turns into something positive. If parents can understand the meaning and the importance of crying, they will be able to value it for what it is and be less afraid of it. So many mothers have said to me, "He's just crying because he wants attention." Right! Correct! And that's okay, because it's what he was programmed to do. Or, as someone who works with me likes to say, "That's his job."

There is a lot of foolishness in the literature about baby cries. I'm often asked questions such as, "How many cries does a baby have? Are there really ten different cries? Eight different cries? Does the baby have one cry for 'I'm hungry,' a different cry for 'I'm wet,' a different cry for 'I'm cold,' or lonely, bored, sick, etc.?"

Of course not. Yes, babies are good at crying, but they're not *that* good. The newborn infant—and here I am talking about your basic healthy, full-term Gerber baby—has two kinds of cries in his songbook. His cry portfolio—his cryfolio—has a basic cry and a pain cry, and they are distinct. They are clearly, audibly different to the human ear whether you are a parent or not, whether it is your baby or not, whether you are male or female, whether you are an adult or a child.

Not surprisingly, the differences between these two kinds of cries show up if you subject the cry sound to acoustical analysis. I can look at an acoustical analysis of a baby's cry—a cryprint—and tell you exactly what kind of cry it is from the way it looks on the printout.

The pain cry is an emergency cry. It is the early warning system, and it means something is really wrong. I remember talking to a mother, years ago, who called to say that her baby had been doing fine but that there had been a sudden change and the baby's cry had become high-pitched. The mother took the baby to the pediatrician, but the baby was fine. Two days later, the baby got a fever and was found to have an infection. In this case, the cry was an early warning sign. The cry changed before the baby had even developed the fever, and his mother was appropriately alert for signs of trouble.

The pain cry is usually high-pitched, loud, and of sudden onset and includes long periods of breath-holding. Often the very first "waaaaah" or burst of this cry is prolonged and then is followed by a long period of breath-holding. Many mothers say that it is the breath-holding that makes them jump up and say, "There's something wrong with my baby." You heard the first "waaaaah" and are waiting for the second. Instead, you hear silence. That's the breath-holding. There's a very scary moment before you hear the second "waaaaah" that lets you know your baby is okay and hasn't stopped breathing—but you still know that something is wrong. When mothers of colicky babies say to me, "He sounds like he's in pain," it is because they are hearing a pain cry.

The other cry in the newborn cryfolio, the basic cry, is used for everything else. It is most typically heard when the baby is hungry, which is why it is often called the hunger cry. It is the same cry the baby uses when her diaper is dirty or for any other nonemergency issue. The basic cry has a more gradual buildup and a lower pitch. It does not have the long periods of breath-holding or the frantic, emergency quality of the pain cry. That's why mothers hearing that cry will often say, "Oh, she's just hungry" or "She just wants to be picked up." They are fairly nonchalant about it, and that's fine.

But all babies are not created equal. In the same way that adult voices are unique, there is a certain individuality to each baby's cry. You see, there is the sound of a sound and there is also the sound inside the sound. The sound of the cry sound is the basic or pain cry. The sound inside the sound—or the cry within the cry—is the unique part of your baby's cry. It is your baby's cry signature. This is why mothers say their baby has a "bored" cry or a "wet" cry. Some babies do develop different kinds of cries within the overall structure of their basic cry that come to have special meaning for their mother. But one baby's "bored" cry is not the same as another's—and not all babies have a "bored" cry.

We also know that some babies have more articulate cries than others. If you think of people you know, you realize that some are more adept at communicating than others, better able to articulate their needs and wants. And think of how important communication is in interpersonal relationships. How often do you hear of marital problems caused by poor communication? Well, just as adults vary in their communication skills, so do babies. Crying is a form of communicative competence. Some babies' cries are just not as clear and well defined as others; their cries may not fit the profile of the "classic" pain cry or basic cry. These are normal babies; they just don't have great communication skills. Their cries may be unusual or different but not abnormal. They are harder to read, and their mothers often say, "I can't tell what he wants."

All of these observations have to do with the newborn to 1-month-old infant. Crying in infants at this age has a reflex quality, as opposed to the more voluntary quality that happens after the first month. At around age 4 to 6 weeks, there are changes in the baby's nervous system that involve the vocal cords and the voice box (the larynx). At that point, the baby starts to gain control of his vocal cords, a prerequisite for speech and language development. (Soon, the baby will coo and babble and start doing all those cute baby things.)

Once the process of voluntary control starts and the baby discovers that she can make sounds when she wants to, her cry is no longer just a reflex. She will still cry for the same reasons she did before, but there is a new dimension now. The baby can initiate the cry. And make no mistake about it, babies love this. It is as if they have discovered a new toy, their first internal toy. And look at the power that comes along with it! "I can make Mommy come whenever I want." Now we have the baby crying for attention, which is different from crying because of hunger or pain.

This is where the battle starts. It is the first time that the baby's will is pitted against the mother's will. Once the attention cry has been added to the baby's cryfolio, once Mom says, "He is doing it on purpose—he just wants attention," the battle line is drawn. When the cry is just from hunger or the baby's needing a diaper change, parents don't feel they have a choice about responding. But once a baby can cry on purpose, parents are faced with their first opportunity to say no. The baby asserts his autonomy—and the challenge begins.

How parents deal with these early issues will set the stage for the relationship they will have with their child for the rest of their lives. When colic is thrown into the equation, that first challenge becomes the first crisis.

CHAPTER TWO

A Visit to the Colic Clinic: Seeking Help in a Crisis

The Colic Clinic is part of the Infant Development Center at Women & Infants Hospital in Providence, Rhode Island. The center is also part of Brown Medical School (check out the center at www.infantdevelopment.org). The center itself is a multidisciplinary group of more than 50 researchers and practitioners. It has both research programs and clinical services, of which the Colic Clinic is one. In addition to treating colic, we offer clinical services for premature infants and their families, for older infants and toddlers with behavior problems, and for infants who are exposed to drugs during pregnancy. We also conduct research programs in these and other areas. I mention all this so that you will understand that we approach colic from a broad and integrated perspective.

There's a lot of back-and-forth between research and services and among the various clinical programs. We learn a lot from one another and our models change as we continue to grow and develop.

We started the Colic Clinic back in the mid-1980s because we were in a bind. We were studying crying and colic and in the process found ourselves giving parents advice and helping them. We found ourselves caught in two worlds: (1) trying to do research, where you can't really focus on treating the individual people you are working with, and (2) providing services. So we split the two components apart, creating a research program and a clinical service so that we could do justice to both.

We see about 75 new patients per year, so we have seen hundreds over the years. Rhode Island is a tiny state: If you drive 30 minutes in any direction, you're in either another state or the ocean. Most of our patients are from Rhode Island, although we have had people travel here from other states. Families are referred to the clinic from the Women & Infants Hospital Warmline, community pediatricians and other physicians, mental health professionals, and families who have been to the clinic. Many times they contact us just because of word of mouth. A mother will call up and say she heard about the clinic from a friend. Some learn about us from the media or from our Web site, www.colic-baby.com.

Babies from all walks of life are carried through the door of our clinic. Most families have insurance, but we also see families without insurance. They come from all kinds of families. Their moms are young and single, or older and married. Some are stay-at-home moms. Some are unemployed. Some are professionals. Some go home to lovely homes on the seashore near here; others live in the projects; some in Providence's older ethnic neighborhoods. Also, we don't see only babies with what is traditionally thought of as colic. Some babies have cry problems because of specific medical conditions such as prematurity or prenatal drug exposure. These babies may have the same kinds of cry problems as babies with colic, but their symptoms are complicated by other medical problems.

All these babies—all these families—have something in common. The babies are unhappy. They're crying, they're not sleeping, their eating patterns are upset. Their moms and dads are upset too. They're sleep deprived. They're discouraged. And they want one thing: They want it to stop!

We have developed a unique model at our clinic. It is really a paradigm shift in that the focus is not on just the baby but on the family as a whole. We view colic as a biopsychosocial issue that involves everyone in the home. It's not just something that is happening to the child. The *bio* in *biopsychosocial* underscores that we are dealing with a biological problem in the infant. The *psychosocial* part is to underscore that impact on the family. We see colic as a problem that can affect the parent–child relationship. Our short-term goal is to prevent the immediate problem from deteriorating into a seriously disordered relationship. Our long-term goal is to give parents the tools to be able to handle problems in the future. (When parents graduate from colic school, they have the tools to deal with other issues as their child grows up).

Because our approach addresses both the medical and behavioral problems of the infant as well as the mental health needs of the family, we consider the mother a patient as well (and it is the mother, in most cases, who approaches us). We recognize that a crying, irritable baby can set up a vicious cycle, in which both baby and Mom—and Dad, too—are miserable. Some 45 percent of the moms who come to us have symptoms of depression. We look to help the whole system of the family, because colic can affect the whole family. We know that colic can lead to sleeping disturbances, feeding problems, difficult temperament, temper tantrums, and behavior problems in the infant. We know that colic can lead to anger and depression in parents, disrupted family relationships, problems in the marriage, and behavior problems in siblings.

We know that colic can alter the way you view your child so that you see her differently, as more vulnerable, as somehow flawed. And if you see her that way, you will treat her that way. We know from school systems how this works. It becomes a self-fulfilling prophecy—if we expect a child to fail, she will fail. The first 3 months of life is a critical period of family development when parents are learning about their children and about their own efficacy as parents. If you have to enroll in colic school, we want to make sure you graduate with honors.

Health care providers need to address maternal functioning and family issues when treating colic in order to make that happen.

When you call the Colic Clinic, Margarita answers the phone. Margarita is from the Dominican Republic, so if your baby is crying in Spanish, we can handle it (only kidding!). Margarita will do a telephone screen to get some sense of what is going on, make sure we are right for you, get you a better referral if we aren't, and set up your intake appointment as soon as possible. Waiting lists are not acceptable for families with colicky babies.

The intake is a way for us to get a history, get some sense of what is going on, and get the ball rolling. When a mother leaves the intake session, she is given a questionnaire packet to fill out at home and bring to the first treatment session. The packet includes the Colic Symptom Checklist (see pages 29–34), a cry diary (see page 28), and questionnaires that tell us about depression, parenting stress, family function, marital satisfaction, maternal self-esteem, and social support.

Treatment at the clinic is brief and intensive and takes place during an important period in infant development. The first few months of life, when colic hits, is a time of rapid change. We watch it, and document it with and for the parents we see. Typically, infants are seen for two to five treatment visits over a 2- to 12-week period—although as with any average, there are exceptions.

The treatment sessions take place in a comfortable room

with a couch that is large enough to accommodate the family. Optimal treatment requires both parents, so we really encourage dads to come as well. Sometimes other family members also come—grandmothers, aunts, the baby's siblings. It can be a real party. And the baby says, "It's my party and I'll cry if I want to." There is also a one-way mirror in the room with an observation room behind it. This is because the clinic is also used for teaching purposes. Medical students rotate through the clinic, and sometimes other guests want to observe. We don't let people observe unless the family gives us permission.

We have two clinicians in the room to provide treatment. One is a behavioral pediatrician. The other is a family support specialist, either a social worker or a psychologist. This is critical and makes our program unique. It may seem like a luxury to have two such high-caliber professionals in the room, but we have found that it is necessary and saves problems in the long run. The treatment is, of course, individualized to the needs of each family. No two families have exactly the same issues and circumstances, although there are common themes. You can be sure they all have crying in common. Feeding and sleeping problems also are common, and the impact on the family is a common issue. It is certainly true that sometimes the predominant problem is medical and sometimes it is psychosocial. But they still affect each other. For example, we may have a baby with GER (gastroesophageal reflux), and you might think, *Oh, that's medical. Treat the baby with medication, "cure" the reflux, and the colic goes away.* It's usually not that simple.

GER happens when contents from the stomach back up into the esophagus, perhaps because a valve in the stomach does not have an effective seal. The stuff of stomachs is often acidic, and it burns. So GER is like infant heartburn. We treat the GER, and it helps with the colic—sometimes—because GER doesn't always cause colic. Our research has confirmed that many babies have some reflux but that it doesn't bother them.

We don't know why colic is related to GER in some babies and not others. What we do know is that having a baby with GER can put a tremendous stress on the family, and that perspective must be addressed as well. I certainly look for signs to see if the balance of treatment is going to be more infant- or parent-focused. When I hear a mother say, "I know what this is. It's colic. I know I didn't cause it," I know there will be much less psychological work than the in the case of the mother who says, "No one can hold this baby but me."

Our treatment sessions usually take a little more than an hour. Toward the end of the session, we develop a set of recommendations in the form of an individualized family treatment plan. (After the treatment session, we also send a follow-up letter to the baby's pediatrician, and we are available for telephone consultation.)

Now that you know the drill, let me introduce you to some of the babies who have been brought here for treatment over the years and have met our staff of physicians, nurses, and mental health professionals. (Details about these children and their parents have been changed to protect their privacy. But these are real babies, with real colic. Believe me. We heard them!)

Amanda was a breast-fed baby. Her mom called the Warmline because the baby didn't sleep through the night. (The Warmline is a free parent-support telephone service at Women & Infants Hospital that offers comfort, support, advice, and referrals to worried parents.) She was up every 15 minutes, all night long. Dad was getting 5 hours of sleep a night; mom was getting 3. Amanda was their first child, born of a planned pregnancy. Her mom, age 30, had been thrilled to be pregnant. But now she wasn't so sure about the result! Her baby pulled away from the nipple during feeds, arching her back as if she felt uncomfortable. She was just not interested in nursing. Instead, she let out "loud, blood-curdling cries," her mom reported.

It turned out that Amanda had significant GER. We recommended some practical fixes: after feeding, her parents were to keep Amanda semireclined for 20 to 30 minutes. They elevated the head of her crib. We told her mom and dad that it was okay to let Amanda cry for 10 to 15 minutes at a time without being picked up. And we prescribed Zantac to reduce stomach acid. To help with breast-feeding, we suggested that her mom stop eating dairy, caffeine, and chocolate. We told her to make the baby's night feedings "business only"—no lights, no play, no stimulation. We suggested a regular bedtime and wake-up time of 7 PM and 7 AM, respectively, and told Mom to put Amanda down for her nap in a consistent place.

And what about Mom and Dad? "Try to make sleep a priority," we told them. Let other things go for the time being. And we suggested that they spend time together as a couple.

Two weeks later, we saw Amanda again. There had been some progress, but the baby was still having trouble with sleeping and feeding. Mom and Dad were still losing sleep, and their marriage was on the back burner. "Try to work time into your schedule to devote to your relationship," we advised. "This is a difficult time physically, and emotionally taxing for both of you. It's not unusual for couples to experience tension in their relationship during such times."

By age 7 months, this baby was pretty much sleeping through the night and was feeding better. She had tried solid foods and was keeping up the Zantac to calm her reflux. In the spring we were able to say, "Congratulations! Amanda is sleeping through the night, transitioning to sleep well, eating well." That was her last visit to the clinic.

Liam was a screamer. He came to us, referred by his pediatrician, at 7 weeks. "He screams all day," his mom told us. She was having a difficult time coping with his extreme amount of crying. The first 5 weeks of her son's life had gone pretty well. Then Liam cried from 8:30 AM to 5:00 PM one day. And he had continued to cry nearly all day every day since then.

Liam's mom was his primary caretaker. His dad had taken

to sleeping in another room to be able to go to work in the morning. Dad told us he had a hard time listening to the crying because he "feels bad for Liam." Liam's mom told us that though she was close to the end of her reserves, she had had no thoughts of harming her baby. She had a support network composed of her mom and a neighbor but was finding it hard to turn to them for help.

We noted on intake that Liam was "inconsolable." He was crying and was clearly a very sensitive, jumpy infant. And 2 weeks later, his mom reported that his crying had improved 75 percent. But his nighttime sleep was still very fragmented. Liam would sleep only in his car seat or in his mom's arms.

By the time he was 10 weeks old, Liam had learned the difference between night and day. He had developed a better sleep pattern—and he slept in his bed, not Mom's arms. Mom and Dad were back in their own bed. They were on the way back to becoming a cheerful family.

Anna's problems took a little longer to resolve. She came to us at age 4 weeks. Her mom, 42, already had two kids. But this one was different. "She cries like she's being tortured," she told us. The baby was at the breast all day. "I feel like a human pacifier," her mom said. The baby calmed down and fell asleep at the breast. Nothing else worked, not car trips, nor the swing, nor the bouncy seat.

Anna had no bedtime routine, we discovered. She was sleeping in her parents' bed. Her diary revealed that this baby cried or fussed 8½ hours, slept 11½ hours, and fed 14 times.

The mom wondered what she would do when she had to return to work.

We told Anna's mom not to allow the baby to fall asleep while nursing. We suggested waiting 2 hours between feedings and not letting the breast serve as a pacifier. We suggested introducing a bottle and letting Dad feed the baby. We told the family to establish a regular bedtime for Anna and to keep her awake for 1½ to 2 hours before it.

We saw Anna next at 2 months. Mom was back to work and was relying less on the breast as a pacifier. She breast-fed Anna when she got home from work. The baby had adjusted well to Mom returning to work; her crying and fussing had decreased. We suggested that Mom nurse for no more than 30 minutes at a time, that she wait 3 hours from one feeding to next, and that she nurse Anna in a quiet place. We prescribed a bedtime routine: a quiet feeding time, lowered lighting, singing a lullaby. The ritual might include listening to a music box or sharing a picture book. The baby should be put in her crib while drowsy but still awake. Infants who know how to fall asleep only while being held have a hard time transitioning back to sleep if they wake up in the middle of the night!

Anthony's mom was at her wit's end when she arrived at the clinic. "Anthony has had a difficult time with feedings from the very start," she told us. We diagnosed maternal depression in this case. Anthony's growth rate had decreased. He cried during feeding. He wasn't sleeping and couldn't soothe himself.

We told his mom, "It's okay to pat Anthony for a couple of minutes before leaving the room when you put him to bed. But remember that you want him to learn to self-soothe and put himself to sleep. If he cries once you leave the room, allow him to cry for 10 to 15 minutes before you go back in. This allows him to learn ways to calm himself down and eventually put himself to sleep. If you feel you must return, use as little interaction as possible. Don't pick him up or turn on the lights."

We also thought this mom was doing way too much parenting on her own. "Allow Dad to give a bottle as the last feeding of the day, after you have retired for the night," we said. "This allows Dad an important and pleasurable role—and gives you a few more precious minutes of sleep."

Two weeks later, we saw Anthony again. Here's what his report said: "Nice work! You have seen a great deal of progress in only 8 days. Anthony is now eating more comfortably (you no longer need to dance with him throughout his bottle). He still wakes in the night, but he's a happier baby during the day now that he is sleeping more. Still fussing up to 4 hours per day. His tiredness is probably part of his irritability. But things are looking up!"

We continued to see Anthony regularly. His sleep still needed attention. "His bedtime routine should end with him in bed drowsy but awake. Start the routine 15 to 30 minutes before sleep time, mostly in his room. Give him his special toy and blanket and a last kiss for the day."

We urged Anthony's mom to find 30 minutes of "mom

time" during the day. We advised her to find a trusted sitter to stay with him on a regular basis, several times a week. We told her to try to nap when the baby did.

This mom, in her depression, was finding herself unable to cope with teaching her infant to regulate himself. Her anxiety and stress and her sleep deprivation made it tough to manage daily routines. She needed daily time alone to take care of herself.

We kept in touch. At 8½ months, there was amazing improvement. Anthony fell asleep with little protest. He napped well in the morning, though he loudly protested afternoon naps. He is happily mobile, crawling and trying to head up the stairs.

We told this mom, "Get a sitter on a *regular* basis. Get out with Anthony now that he is happier and more social. Keep up your half-hour of mom time. And get out as a couple before your next visit."

We saw Anthony again when he was 2½. He is still a picky eater, but he is a cheerful kid. He still fights bedtime and naptime and has tantrums sometimes. His parents are happier and are very supportive of each other—but they're still exhausted. Depression remains an issue for Mom, and the family has a new baby girl in the house in addition to Anthony. Though he's much better, Anthony has persistent sleep problems. He has night terrors sometimes. His family's file with us remains open.

As you can see from these stories, parenting a colicky child is tough. And as a culture, we don't prepare our parents for it in advance. Colic is isolating, disturbing, frustrating, and exhausting. It wreaks havoc with your self-esteem and impacts your marriage. It gets between you and your baby. But it can be managed, as these moms and dads learned.

Without treatment, colic can affect your relationship with your child long after the crying stops. Figuring it out can make a huge difference. Let me end this chapter with a quote from a letter we received from a mom whose daughter we treated at the clinic. We keep this letter tacked up on the bulletin board in our waiting room, along with all the pictures of smiling infants and toddlers that parents send us. We think this letter probably gives some of the nervous parents sitting in our waiting room some hope:

> Katie has become a joy and we are becoming a family again now that we are no longer controlled by Katie's physical conditions. All my fears and concerns of being unable to bond with Katie were for nothing as I love her with all my heart. Each time she looks at me with that smile and those twinkling eyes it pushes all those dark memories further away. I tolerate her cries now with ease. No knee-jerk reaction, none of that pit-of-my-stomach feelings at the first whimper. I know now that there is life after colic.

COLIC TOOLS

If you're wondering how much your baby is crying and whether your baby has colic, here are two tools that we use. The diary divides each 24-hour day into 15-minute sections, each with check boxes for if the child is crying, sleeping, feeding, and/or awake. At the end of every week, highlight the four behaviors in four different colors. This lets you see how much your child is actually crying, and when it is most likely to occur—and gives you a better sense of control and a clearer view of the situation. It also shows you when your child is *not* crying and what else he is doing. It might help you take advantage of the awake times so that you know when the baby is available for some good "quality time." The Colic Symptom Checklist will help you see whether your baby has colic symptoms in addition to excessive crying.

Cry Diary

During each 15-minute period of the day, you are to indicate the main activity of your baby. The baby behaviors you will record are F=fussing, C=crying, S=sleeping, E=eating, A=awake.

Month	Day	Year

12 MN ☐☐☐☐ **1 AM** ☐☐☐☐ **2 AM** ☐☐☐☐ **3 AM** ☐☐☐☐

4 AM ☐☐☐☐ **5 AM** ☐☐☐☐ **6 AM** ☐☐☐☐ **7 AM** ☐☐☐☐

8 AM ☐☐☐☐ **9 AM** ☐☐☐☐ **10 AM** ☐☐☐☐ **11 AM** ☐☐☐☐

12 NOON ☐☐☐☐ **1 PM** ☐☐☐☐ **2 PM** ☐☐☐☐ **3 PM** ☐☐☐☐

4 PM ☐☐☐☐ **5 PM** ☐☐☐☐ **6 PM** ☐☐☐☐ **7 PM** ☐☐☐☐

8 PM ☐☐☐☐ **9 PM** ☐☐☐☐ **10 PM** ☐☐☐☐ **11 PM** ☐☐☐☐

Where baby falls asleep (S=swing, A=arms, B=parents' bed, Ba=bassinette, C=crib, CS=car seat)–place above the block designating onset of a sleep episode.

Best 5 minutes of the day: _____

Total hours: Fussing ___ Crying ___ Sleeping ___ Awake ___ Eating ___

Colic Symptom Checklist

PART I: CRYING HISTORY

1. How many hours in a typical day does your
   baby cry or fuss?   _____ HRS/DAY

2. Does your baby ever cry or fuss, more than
   3 hours in a day?   _____ YES _____ NO

3. How many days per week does your baby cry
   for more than 3 hours per day?   _____ DAYS

4. How many weeks old was your baby when the
   colic or extreme crying began?   _____ WEEKS

5. How many weeks did your baby cry for more
   than 3 hours or have problems with
   extreme crying?   _____ WEEKS

6. How did you decide the crying was colic?
   ____ Pediatrician diagnosed
   ____ Advice from friends
   ____ Reading
   ____ Previous experience with a colicky baby
   ____ By the baby's behavior

PART II: CRYING EPISODES

	Y	N
7. Does your baby fuss or cry throughout most of the day?	☐	☐
8. Does your baby have crying episodes that are different or seem to come "out of the blue"?	☐	☐

9. Do these crying episodes usually

	Y	N
a. Occur suddenly	☐	☐
b. Gradually build up?	☐	☐
c. *Seem unpredictable?*	☐	☐

10. Just before the crying episodes, is your baby *usually*:

____ Fussing or crying?

____ Happy?

____ In no particular mood or state?

____ Other (specify: _____)

11. Is there anything that occurs just before the crying episode?

____ Feeding

____ Sleeping

____ Loud noises/disruption

____ No consistent pattern

____ Other (specify:_____)

12. How would you describe the crying episodes?

_____

13. What typically happens after the episode ends?

____ Baby continues to fuss or cry

____ Baby eats

____ Baby sleeps

____ Baby is awake and content

____ No consistent pattern

____ Other (specify: _____)

PART III: CRY QUALITY

14. What does your baby's cry sound like during a crying episode?
    (Check all that apply.)

____ High pitch	____ Pain
____ Loud	____ Top of the lungs
____ Intense	____ Scream
____ Abnormal	____ Sick
____ Irritating	____ Annoying
____ Other (specify:_____)	

15. Is the cry during an episode different than the crying that occurs at
    other times of the day?

____ Yes. *How* is it different? _____

____ No

PART IV: CRYING IN ACTION

16. What does your baby *look like* during one of these episodes? (Check all that apply,)

____ Hands/fists clenched	____ Holding breath
____ Stomach tight or hard	____ Legs stiff
____ Elbows flexed	____ Arched back
____ Arms stiff	____ Legs, knees drawn up
____ Very active	____ Face red
____ Feet cold	____ Blue or pale around the mouth

PART V: SOOTHING

17. How difficult is it in general to calm your baby during an episode of colic?

____ Very easy: calms immediately

____ Easy: calms after a minute or two

____ Variable: sometimes calms quickly, sometimes cannot be calmed

____ Difficult: takes more than a few minutes and more than minimal effort to calm

____ Very difficult: takes more than several minutes and a lot of effort to calm

____ Inconsolable: crying lasts more than several minutes and nothing calms her/him

18. How does your baby generally act when you are trying to calm him or her?

____ Is soothed by my attempts to calm him or her

____ Is not affected by my attempts to calm him or her

____ My attempts at soothing make him or her cry more

____ My baby resists my attempts to soothe him or her by arching the back or struggling with me

19. Have you given your baby any medications for colic?

____ Yes; list _____

____ No

20. Have you noticed any improvement after giving your baby medication?

____ Yes

____ No

21. Place an X in the boxes next to the things you have *tried and* the things that have been *successful* for calming your baby:

a. Leave baby alone	☐ TRIED	☐ SUCCESSFUL
b. Talk to the baby	☐ TRIED	☐ SUCCESSFUL
c. Sound or music	☐ TRIED	☐ SUCCESSFUL
d. Put the baby on his/her belly	☐ TRIED	☐ SUCCESSFUL
e. Pat the baby	☐ TRIED	☐ SUCCESSFUL
f. Stroke the baby	☐ TRIED	☐ SUCCESSFUL
g. Rub or massage	☐ TRIED	☐ SUCCESSFUL
h. Pacifier	☐ TRIED	☐ SUCCESSFUL
i. Feed	☐ TRIED	☐ SUCCESSFUL

j. Change diaper   ☐ TRIED   ☐ SUCCESSFUL

k. Swaddle   ☐ TRIED   ☐ SUCCESSFUL

l. Hold in arms   ☐ TRIED   ☐ SUCCESSFUL

m. Hold on shoulder   ☐ TRIED   ☐ SUCCESSFUL

n. Hold upright   ☐ TRIED   ☐ SUCCESSFUL

o. Rock   ☐ TRIED   ☐ SUCCESSFUL

p. Bounce   ☐ TRIED   ☐ SUCCESSFUL

q. Walk with   ☐ TRIED   ☐ SUCCESSFUL

r. Swing   ☐ TRIED   ☐ SUCCESSFUL

s. Car ride   ☐ TRIED   ☐ SUCCESSFUL

t. Vibration device/washer/dryer   ☐ TRIED   ☐ SUCCESSFUL

u. Other; list: _____   ☐ TRIED   ☐ SUCCESSFUL

CHAPTER THREE

The Crying Game: Negotiating Your Relationship with Your Baby

rying is not a game in the sense of an activity or pastime. When your baby cries, she's not doing it for amusement. Crying is a game in the sense that it's a contest, a match that involves struggle and a strategy for gaining a desired end. And the crying game has its own set of rules.

Crying involves matches—and mismatches—between infants and their mothers. Part of the strategy for winning the crying game involves changing mismatches into matches. The goal is what we child development folks call "goodness of fit." A good fit happens when an infant's and a mother's characteristics match. (And by a *good fit*, I don't mean a particularly rousing version of one of your baby's crying fits.) Good fit is the cornerstone for developing a healthy relationship with your baby. Achieving a good fit is something we help parents with at the Colic Clinic.

It is important to understand that colic can cause a disturbance—a perturbation—in the baby–parent relationship Whether a baby's crying is related to feeding, temperament, or anything else, it still changes the parent–child relationship. I suspect you already know that, or you would not be reading this. It's a natural worry for parents of colicky babies—so let's get it out on the table.

What do I mean by disturbance or perturbation? In infant psychiatry, we talk about differences between relationship disturbances or perturbations and relationship disorders. (I love the image of a baby lying on the couch, with the therapist sitting on a chair behind the baby's head and holding a notepad.) What's the difference between a disturbance and a disorder? A disturbance is basically a bump in the road, a deviation that is part of the normal developmental process. A disorder, on the other hand, means psychopathology, or vulnerability.

In most cases, colic is—or at least starts out as—a "disturbance in the field." It causes a change in the developing parent–child relationship. The relationship becomes derailed and is temporarily off track. It goes without saying that this is not a positive development, although we will see that it can lead to positive resolution and positive changes later on. (Yes, there is light at the end of the tunnel—as long as you don't have tunnel vision.) A disturbance happens within normal limits, and you will find that child rearing is full of these speed bumps. In fact, much of parenting could be described as negotiating bumps in the road, followed by corrections, just as when you slow down and grab the steering wheel when you're driving. The cycle repeats itself throughout the life span: bump → correction → bump → correction. The bumps are unavoidable, but it is how you make the correction—or what Dr. Edward Tronick calls the repair process—that makes the difference.

You can see where I'm going with this, can't you? This is parenting, not rocket science. Did you ever wonder why there are many more parents than rocket scientists? Parenting is something we can all do, and we almost always do well. So let's give ourselves a break. I am not underestimating how hard it is to parent. But I do want to acknowledge that we all have natural abilities in this area—Dr. Hanus Papousek called it "intuitive parenting." If we trusted our intuition, we would probably realize that we know more than we think we know. What happens if the correction after the bump fails? We run the risk of shifting from a slight jolt to an accident—from a relationship disturbance to a relationship disorder. In other words, to psychopathology—an abnormal and potentially dangerous situation. Even if that happens, we are still not talking doomsday, but a disorder is harder to fix than a disturbance. So why let it get that far? If we intervene early, we can prevent a relationship disturbance from becoming a relationship disorder and prevent psychopathology in the parent–child relationship.

Here is an example: One winter, I was getting ready to board an airplane for an all-night flight. Also boarding was a mother carrying a screaming baby. My gut told me before my brain did that something was wrong. The mother was holding the baby straight out in front of her, as if he were lying on a board, and rocking him by moving her arms up and down. The baby looked uncomfortable, and so did the mother. I wanted to go over, take the baby, and put him upright on my shoulder. As the mother was getting on the plane, I could see the look in the passengers' eyes saying, *Please—not in my cabin, not near me!*

The baby continued his loud, high-pitched screaming through taxi and takeoff and for what seemed like another hour. The mother never changed his position, although she periodically tried to bottle-feed him. She was sitting about five rows in front of me. The other passengers were ready to kill her!

Then it stopped. I think you could actually feel a change in cabin pressure from the collective sigh of relief from the passengers. I knew the mom was standing in one of the corridors, and I had to see what was going on. So I got up and watched. The baby was sound asleep in that same horizontal position. He had probably just worn himself out. Then I saw the mother shift the baby to her left arm and with her right hand take out a bottle. The alarms were going off in my head: *No! Please! Don't! You finally got the kid to sleep. Why would you do this?*

Sure enough, she stuck the bottle in the sleeping kid's mouth, he startled, woke, spat the nipple out—and started screaming again. It went on for another good half hour. There was a good chance that that baby had colic. And his crying had escalated into a failing or already failed relationship with his mother.

Understanding colic is so important—and is the reason I do what I do—because for many parents colic is the first bump in the road. It would be a simplistic exaggeration to say that colic is going to determine or ruin your relationship with your child forever. Yet because it is the first disturbance, it will influence how you deal with the second disturbance, the third, and so on, creating a template for how you deal with future interactions with your child.

After colic, because of what you have been through, your relationship with your baby will be different. Not necessarily worse. Not necessarily better—but different. You will have learned from the experience. You will carry your new relationship with your baby and the lessons you learned forward into the post-colic era—into the "aftercry." Colic changes you. It changes how see your baby, how you react to, perceive, and feel about your baby forever. I know this is true because of the stories I have heard over the years from parents who had colicky babies. It is almost as if the aftercry never ends.

Mothers who had colicky babies have very strong feelings about the experience. They talk about colic with great intensity and have incredibly vivid memories of the details, whether the colic was 2 years or 32 years ago. These mothers sound as if they had been through a trauma—not the kind that makes you forget but the kind that makes you want, and need, to tell it over and over again.

Why is the memory of colic so powerful? Because it is unresolved. The babies may have stopped crying, but the mothers are still trying to figure out the experience, put the pieces back together, put themselves back together, and understand the magnitude of the ordeal. Even years later, the experience remains unsettled. It gnaws at them, and they will tell their story to anyone who will listen. Ultimately, and tragically, they are still asking, "What did I do wrong?" They haven't forgiven themselves, and they're not even sure what they should be forgiven for. They just feel like they did something wrong. If there is something wrong with their child, they blame it on the colic that they "caused." I have heard colic blamed for everything from attention-deficit hyperactivity disorder to autism, but what is most striking to me is the intensity and clarity with which the experience comes back into memory— as if the mothers can call it up and relive it at will.

Another part of what makes colic so devastating, and I mean psychologically devastating to parents, is that you get blindsided. You don't see it coming. As one mother in the colic clinic said to me, "I put an angel to bed, and the child from hell woke up." Part of why the relationship goes off track is because you feel like you've been hit by a train. Your hopes, dreams, and fantasies about the perfect baby have been ruined. Overnight.

It's not only about your fears of having a colicky baby. It's your fears about yourself. For many, having a colicky baby confirms their worst fears about their competence as parents. A mother might think, *This is my fault. I knew it. I knew I couldn't do this.*

It doesn't always happen this way. Not all colic comes out of the blue, and not all mothers blame themselves. There are many pathways and reactions to having a colicky baby.

The story line that involves colic coming out of the blue—the overnight exploder—is real. I wish I could tell you what percentage of colicky babies it represents, but I can't. While it's not the only story line, it is important because it represents a sudden, unexpected violation.

Think about it. You take home your gorgeous new baby. He does all the things that you expected and hoped for during the first 4 to 5 weeks. You're doing it. You're being a parent! You didn't screw up. He eats, he sleeps (maybe not through the night, but he's getting there). You can see progress. He is becoming more alert, sociable, and playful during the day. You even laugh when he pees in your face. You laugh harder when he pees in his dad's face. You are sleep-deprived, putting in long days as a mother, and maybe it is more demanding than you thought, but at some level you knew it would be like this. You read the books. You heard the stories—your friends, mother, and mother-in-law told you all about it. Secretly, you are starting to feel pretty good about yourself. It's only been a few weeks, but your baby is growing, and he's cute as hell, and you love him to death, and you are starting to feel like a competent (can you admit it to yourself?) mother.

As your baby becomes more and more alert, he looks you in the eyes and you melt. You are getting something back from him. And you can't wait to see that 6-week smile. After all your hard work, you're even starting to feel that you deserve these goodies. This whole mother–baby relationship is being primed for success. In Yiddish, there is the word *qvell*, which describes that warmest of feelings inside your heart that is more than pride. When your baby looks at you, you feel so good that you almost want to burst into tears.

It is such an unkind setup because instead of that 6-week smile, you get the screaming meanie from hell. No wonder you feel like you've been hit by a train. You're devastated, overcome by conflicting emotions. You are concerned about your baby because he seems to be suffering and in pain. He is screaming, and you feel helpless. You can't stop the crying. Overnight, you feel inadequate as a mother. You are disappointed and angry and feel almost violated. You feel guilty for being angry. Some of your anger may be directed at your baby. More guilt. You feel responsible. After all, you are the mother. And then you start wondering if you can handle this. You have fears about hurting your baby. More guilt. Fears about the long-term consequences. Fears about what this is going to do to your family. Will your husband/mother/mother-in-law blame you? What will your friends say? You have failed your first test as a new mom. Where do you go from here? How do you pick up the pieces? How do you get back on track?

This is why colic is so important. It's not just the crying. Your pediatrician is right. The crying will stop. But the real trick is how to repair your relationship with your baby to prevent a downward spiral into psychopathology. You need to get back to normal, restore your self-esteem, and learn from this experience so that you are better prepared for the next bump in the road. If you do, then when your teenager walks in the house with a ring in his nose and another in his belly button, you'll be able to say to yourself, *I know this feeling. I've been here before, and I'll get through this.*

The "exploder" is not the only kind of colicky baby. Another common colic scenario, or pathway, involves the baby that I think of as "the escalator." A gradual buildup pathway, escalation is not as dramatic, but it's just as problematic. This kid cries a little more the older she gets, until the crying is enough for the baby to earn her colic label. Obviously, with an escalator the parents are spared the shock faced by the parents of an exploder, but these parents face a different kind of relationship challenge. Escalators are often persistently cranky babies. They may not cry a lot, but they are fussy and irritable practically all the time. Unlike the exploders, who may have a good first month, the escalators are often miserable from the get-go. They don't cry enough to be called colicky (the colic label is usually not applied until a baby is at least a few weeks old anyway), but the parent–child relationship never really gets off to a positive start. You never get the goodies—the alertness, the social interaction, the playfulness. Even constant attention doesn't keep the baby from being miserable. The only good part comes when the baby is sleeping, so your "reward" is not having to be with your baby. This is not what you bargained for, and it makes you feel incredibly inadequate from the beginning. There is little reinforcement for being a good mother in this scenario, so it is easy for these mothers to blame themselves. My impression is that mothers of "escalators" are most prone to depression—and it is easy to see why.

The notion of "goodness of fit" is probably the single most important construct for understanding how to deal with crying and colic—and how to deal with parenting in general, for that matter. Here's how it works: The interaction between infant and mother as the pair works out a relationship is a dance. There is back and forth and rhythm and cadence and reciprocity and coming together and flying apart. It takes two to tango—but it takes only one to cry. And what happens when you are learning to dance? You step on each other's toes. Then you correct. Repair. And that is exactly what mothers and babies do with each other. They are trying to work out a relationship, define boundaries, and see what works and what doesn't work.

The relationship is also a bargaining table. We talk about "developing" relationships, but this is not how it works between mothers and babies, any more than between adults. We don't develop relationships, we *negotiate* them. You're probably thinking, *How do you negotiate with a baby? Babies don't talk or listen to reason.* Well, if you've gotten this far in the book, you're a little more crylingual than that. You know that babies do talk. They have a language. Their cry and their behavior is their language, and parents can learn how to understand a baby's language and have a conversation.

Each partner brings his or her own stuff—issues—to the bargaining table in a relationship. In the case of mothers, these issues are characteristics, personality, feelings, behaviors, expectations, and fantasies. In the case of babies, they are behaviors, reactions, physical characteristics, and what some call temperament (what later becomes personality). Negotiating a relationship demands a great deal of back and forth and give and take as each partner looks for his or her comfort zone (or cry zone). Like any good relationship, the parent–child connection is dynamic.

Sometimes I worry that we focus too much on the baby's needs and not enough on the needs of the parents. This might sound like heresy, especially from a "baby person" like me, but there are times when the needs of babies and parents are mutually exclusive. We all know that there is abuse and neglect and shaken baby syndrome, but these are the exceptions. The majority of parents are trying to make it with their baby. Their motivation is to do right by their baby.

But what happens when the baby's needs and the parent's

needs conflict? You are put in what family therapist and author Dr. David Schnarch calls the crucible. You have a conflict. You are being tested. You have to make a choice. And, in most cases, what to do is the real issue. More important for the parents is the process, the feelings involved, and the aftermath. You *will* pick up, soothe, walk around with, and change the baby (and I don't mean change the baby for a different baby, although you might want to do that too). You *will* get up in the middle of the night and stumble around in a sleepless daze for days, weeks, or months. You *will* do all of these PC (in this case, "parentally correct") things because your motivation is where it should be. You are a caring, loving parent who wants to do the best for your baby. What's missing from this equation is you. How do you feel about it? What is the cost to you personally? What about your needs? What happens when your needs are not being met? And if the baby is the bottom line, how do you keep from passing the costs back to your relationship with your baby?

It is hard to take care of someone else when your own needs are not being met. Some of the most difficult cases we have seen at the colic clinic are those involving a depressed mother and a colicky baby. How can you take care of a screaming baby when you yourself are depressed? Where do you even get the energy to get up in the morning? To function? It is remarkable to me, and a real testimonial to these mothers, that they do as well as they do and that they know enough to get help. Of course I worry about the mothers who don't get help, and I know they're out there.

The key principle in the parent–child relationship is goodness of fit. It is based on the concept of matching, in which the characteristics, including expectations, of one partner are in line with the characteristics of the other, and mismatching, in which the characteristics of the two partners are in conflict. With colic, the dramatic change in the baby throws the match out of balance. The mother and baby I saw on the plane were a classic mismatch. When we treat the colic, we also aim to get the relationship back on an even keel. To make this happen, both the baby and the parents need to change.

All kinds of mismatches take place in parenting babies. A baby may cry for only 1 hour a day, but even that drives the mother nuts. Her pediatrician tells her that 1 hour a day of crying is normal and that the baby does not have colic. She should just deal with it! But the mismatch causes a problem in the relationship. The mother has to deal with the fact that she can't stand her baby's crying, and because she has been told that her baby is fine, she will probably conclude that there is something wrong with her.

Another mother I saw had a 3-month-old, calm, beautiful baby who rarely cried and was very sociable. The mom was worried that he was a blob, and she was waiting for the other shoe to drop. She feared that he was brain-damaged, though he was not. That's a mismatch, too.

Because relationships are not static, goodness of fit is a dynamic concept. For babies, that means growth, behavior, and development. Parenting is a series of alignments, misalignments, and realignments as we go in and out of matches and mismatches as the baby changes and parents change.

How do parents change? Parents change because their feeling, attitudes, and even competencies change as babies change. Some parents feel that they can't communicate with a baby until she talks. Talking brings the child's characteristics in line with the parent's characteristics. With language, they can relate and are a better fit. Relationships are also dynamic because of the concept of reciprocity. Each partner modifies the behavior of the other in a constantly changing fashion. They shape each other through mutual feedback. It is an ongoing, fluid system, and you can enter it at any point. Mother reacts to baby, which causes a different reaction in the baby, which in turn changes the way the mother reacts to the baby, each modifying the other in constant, dynamic feedback.

I'm going to let you in on something that I believe but can't prove: I believe that there is an evolutionary purpose to these interactions. I believe there is a driving force that pushes the mother–baby system in the right direction, and that the force comes from within both the baby and the mother. In short, mothers mostly know what they are doing. That's intuitive parenting. Sometimes situations like colic happen to throw us off track. In some cases we need a little help, but in most cases we get back on the train.

Now you understand the crying game. It's a game for life. The stakes are high. But when you look at your baby, you know there is no better payoff.

CHAPTER FOUR

A Colic Case Study: "Bring me a baby who doesn't cry"

I f you have been reading this book in your house with your colicky baby, you are probably feeling isolated and alone. You may be feeling like an inadequate mom, wondering if you're the only mother in America whose baby won't stop crying.

Take it from me: You are not alone. Let's meet a patient from our clinic and hear her story in her own words. Stacy (names and identifying details have been changed to protect privacy), age 32, is the mother of two. She works as a para-legal; husband Greg is a police officer in their hometown. They live in the neighborhood where they grew up, close to extended family and lifelong friends. Son Michael was 4½ when his sister Rachel arrived. Michael didn't have colic, so when Rachel started to fuss it came as a complete surprise.

"It started when she was thirteen days old," Stacy says. "She was the perfect child between zero days and twelve days. She napped and she slept and she was appropriately cuddly. She didn't cry; she didn't spit up. And then on day thirteen, she started crying.

"I came out of the hospital so confident. She was nursing beautifully. I thought I was a great mom, and this is going to be such a fun adventure, and we're a complete family of four. And then day thirteen arrived and threw it into chaos."

Stacy didn't know what was wrong.

"I thought she was in pain. When it got bad over the next few days, she would be so rigid that she couldn't catch her breath. You could stand her up and hold her with one finger and she would stay there. It was horrible. I would put her to the breast and it would be 'Get away from me!' It was scream, suck suck, scream suck suck, scream. I went through the whole 'She hates me, she's allergic to my milk, she hates me' thing."

Like most moms in her situation, Stacy turned to her pediatrician for help. Now, I'm not saying she didn't have a good doctor. But the fact is that many pediatricians know very little about how to deal with colic—and with what we call "colic moms"—as Stacy discovered.

"Before I had Rachel, I would have said that my pediatrician was the best pediatrician in the world," she says. "But I don't think he was equipped to deal with this. I called every day for two weeks saying, 'Something is desperately wrong,' and he said, 'She has colic.'

"'What do I do?' I wanted to know. I wanted to pool our resources and get a plan and then work that plan. And he was, like, 'Oh, she'll get over it.'"

It's true that Rachel will get over colic. But hearing that—which is hard to believe when you're in the middle of the storm—was no help to Stacy in dealing with the here and now.

"I wasn't getting a lot of sympathy," she says. "But I didn't want sympathy. I wanted a plan. I wanted to know what I could do."

Stacy's son Michael had just started preschool when Rachel's colic hit. She turned from her pediatrician to the mommy network at her son's school for help. "I told one mom there about Rachel. And she said, try Zantac. So I asked my doctor and he wrote me out a prescription. And it had a marginal effect. Then I tried stopping nursing and put her on Nutragamen. On the first day, it seemed like it was the answer. But three days later she was crying again."

As Stacy tells her story, her eyes fill with tears repeatedly—although Rachel's colic is now in the past. The intensity, the power, of the experience remains very close to the surface.

"Rachel was crying, and I was crying, but I didn't have postpartum depression, but after three weeks of crying and screaming—well, it's a long day." Baby Rachel screamed all day and slept all night, Stacy recalls. "So I was not sleep deprived. But I was crying, too."

Before Rachel was born, Stacy had purchased a baby sling for carrying her around. At first, Greg objected to the sling, feeling it kept the baby away from him. "The day we came home from the hospital, I came downstairs and I'm wearing her—she's slung way down on my hip—and my husband says, 'I'm not into that sling. That's just another way for her to bond to you and not to me. I'm not using that thing.' But day thirteen, when she started crying, let me tell you, he was saying, 'Can I get you the sling? Can I wash the sling? Because when I put her in the sling, she calmed down. I called her my little joey because she was like a little kangaroo baby back in the pouch. I could rig it so she could see out or I could rig it so she was right up against me. Five minutes of walking around with that and she was done crying."

Even 4½-year-old Michael got the message. "He had a certain expectation of how life was supposed to be," Stacy says of her son. "He was not happy with this screamer. It got to the point where Michael would scream, 'Sling her up! Sling her up!'"

One of the things that is hardest for other people to understand about having a colicky baby—which you know if you have one—is its relentlessness. Stacy pauses in her story, looks down, and speaks softly at this memory.

"I had a low point," she says. "Friends were having a

Christmas party, and the baby was just a bitch all day long. I just didn't know what to do. Even the sling wasn't helping that day. I was frazzled. My husband was at work and my son was at a friend's house. The only thing that was getting me through was that I was going to that Christmas party. I was thinking, there are going to be women there who are going to want to hold this baby, and I am going to sit down and have a meal.

"Well, man plans and God laughs," Stacy says. "We got to the party and she escalated. Maybe it was the busyness or the smells at the party. Who knows why. So I went in to a bedroom and tried to nurse her. She was rejecting me. Now, in my mind she is the biggest distraction in the world, she's ruining everybody's day. In reality she was only ruining my day. My friends felt bad for me." Stacy begins to cry.

"They wanted to have me stay, but I said, 'No, I've got to get her home. I've got to go.' I told my husband he should stay, that one of us should enjoy the holiday. I drove around for a while to see if she would fall asleep—she didn't—so I went home."

Stacy's voice lowers as she tells this part of her story.

"After an hour, I am rocking her and I'm burping her, I'm patting her back and I'm burping her. And then I'm burping her harder and harder. And then I put her down on the bed, not very gently, and I call my husband and I say, 'You need to come home now. You need to come home right now.' Then I sat in the chair and watched her cry.

"When he got home he picked her up and said, 'What do

you want me to do?'" Stacy is crying harder as she tells her story. "And I said, 'I want you to take her away and bring me a baby who doesn't cry.' And he stepped up. For two days, he could soothe her and he could calm her. When I needed him to be there, he was totally there."

After this crisis, Stacy decided to seek help again. She called the Warmline. She asked for a lactation consultant, because she thought she was nursing wrong, and that was causing Rachel's crying. "I called her, but I was too emotional to talk to her," Stacy says. Greg talked with the consultant, and she directed the family to the Colic Clinic, where Rachel was examined and observed.

"The doctor there said, 'Okay, here's the deal. Your daughter does have colic. And you need to get her out of that sling because she's not sleeping during the day. And here's what you're going to do: You're also going to let that child cry in somebody else's arms, and you and your husband are going to go out.'"

The advice sounded difficult to follow, but practical, action-oriented Stacy was willing to give it a try. "They gave me a strategy. They gave me a plan. They gave me a diary. They told me I had to give up the sling because she wasn't learning how to do things. And I did it. I got her out of the sling. I got her to take two naps, even though it was just an hour a day. And I called the clinic and reported, 'She is only sleeping an hour each time.' The doctor said, 'What are you complaining about?' It was one of the first times I laughed, I think. I found out I wasn't crazy. Someone said, 'Yes, your daughter is miserable, and this is what's wrong with her. And yes, it is going to end. But here are some strategies that we're going to give you to get through in the meantime.'"

Stacy slowly put the clinic's suggestions into effect, and tensions eased in her household. Stacy says that husband Greg will "tell anyone who'll listen, 'When my wife came home from that colic clinic she was literally a different person. It was like the weight of the world was lifted off my shoulders.'"

About 6 weeks later, Stacy recalls, she took Rachel over to visit her grandmother. "I took the baby over to my mom's and I said, 'I'm just going to go for a walk around the block.' And my mom said, 'You know, every time I touch her, she cries.' And I said, 'Every time *I* touch her, she cries. You can do this for an hour. I have to do this for twenty-four.'"

Stacy's story shows how colic affects not just the mom-and-baby dyad but the whole family—Mom, Dad, siblings, and the extended family—as well.

Feeling more confident as she followed our clinic's advice, Stacy started making time for herself—and taking proactive steps to make life easier for Rachel too. She started working out at the Y, which offers child care. "I would drop her off with a big note that said, 'Hi. My name is Rachel and I have colic. These are the things that you can try. I like to be held. But if it doesn't work, come and get Mommy, and we'll try it next time.'

"Once I went to the clinic, I no longer felt like I was out

there in the desert wandering with a screaming infant. And early on, it did feel like that. And it defined who she was. She wasn't a lovable baby. She was a screaming monster baby. You love them anyway—but you can't stand them. It's not what you picture during your nine months of miserable pregnancy."

By the time Rachel was almost 5 months old, her crying, and the family's trial, was over. "She became a user-friendly baby," Stacy says, but the memory of the screaming-meemies phase is vivid.

"There were few happy moments," she says. "And I can honestly say that I would not go back to the beginning for all the tea in China. People say, 'Oh, I wish my babies could stay young.' And I say, 'No, no, no.'"

CHAPTER FIVE

Colic Defined:
The Rule of Three Is
Not for Me

"So what is colic?" This and "How many different cries does a baby have?" are the two questions I am most frequently asked. What parents really want to know is: What causes colic, and how is colic defined and diagnosed? How can I make it go away? Underlying all the questions is the biggie: Is it my fault? The answers are more complicated than you might think.

We still don't know what causes colic. There is no simple cure, no magic bullet, to make the baby stop crying. And despite many heroic attempts by pediatricians and researchers to downplay the condition, the suffering of colicky babies and their parents goes on daily. Colic makes professionals feel incompetent because they can't treat something that upsets families so much.

Despite what many well-meaning pediatricians tell their patients, colic is not a harmless condition. Our research—as well as plenty of others'—has shown that these babies are more likely to have difficult temperaments and to experience feeding and sleeping problems. Their cries and their heart rates are different. How the family functions can be impaired. Their parents perceive them as more vulnerable. They can go on to have behavior issues in preschool and problems later on in school with attention/hyperactivity, sensory integration, and emotional reactivity.

You don't have to know what causes colic to be able to recognize, define, or diagnose it. There is a traditional definition of colic called the Rule of Three that is probably the one pediatricians use most. Developed in 1954 by pediatrician Morris Wessel, it was based on the patients that he was seeing in his practice in New Haven, Connecticut. I don't like it much, but in all fairness, it has been around for a long time. Here it is: The Rule of Three says that colic exists when an otherwise normal, healthy baby cries for at least 3 hours a day for at least 3 days a week and has been doing this for at least 3 weeks.

One problem with this definition is that it equates colic with excessive crying, and it explains why the literature often uses phrases such as "colic or excessive crying." As we explained in chapter 1, normally developing babies increase the amount they cry over the first 6 weeks. About 20 percent of babies cry for 3 hours a day or more—and that has been fairly well established. Babies who cry 3 hours a day may not have colic but may simply be normal babies with difficult temperaments.

There may indeed be babies who cry excessively because of colic—but there is more to colic than excessive crying. For many colicky babies there is a distinct colic episode. The baby has normal periods of crying during the day, but when he reaches a colicky phase, there is something different going on. Mothers say all the time: "This is not his normal crying, this is colic." For many babies, this period happens in the early evening. There's even an article in the scientific literature entitled "Early Evening Colic." The point is that regardless of when it occurs—and it does not occur in all colicky babies—there is a separate, distinct period and it has an episodic quality about it.

Many babies with colic have additional symptoms that occur especially during this distinct colic episode. At the Colic Clinic, we group these symptoms into four areas. In fact, our Colic Symptom Checklist (see chapter 2, pages 29–34), is a published instrument and has been used by us and by others to identify these symptoms.

The main source for the symptoms, behaviors, and characteristics on the checklist come from the parents I've seen at the clinic and from countless interviews, magazine articles, and desperate calls and e-mails to friends and family. The second source was the scientific literature. What I learned from the research studies was that not all babies show all character-istics and not all babies show the same characteristics. But most show some. The four characteristics are sudden onset, cry quality, physical signs, and inconsolability.

Let's take a closer look at the four characteristics: *Sudden onset* means that the colic episode seems to come out of the blue. One mother described it by saying, "It's as if my baby is possessed." Another term for this is *paroxysmal onset*, which suggests the sudden and episodic quality that sets it apart from regular crying. It is as if the baby is separated or insulated from the outside world. The episode takes on a life of its own. You get the feeling that this is something that is going to have to run its course. While you may be able to dampen it or ease it somewhat, you can't really stop it. What you have to do is ride it out and make the baby—and yourself—as comfortable as possible.

The second characteristic is the cry quality. The cry changes—not in the same way for all babies, but for most ba-bies there is a qualitative change in the cry during an episode. For many babies, the cry takes on the characteristics of pain cry. Mothers say that their babies sound as if they're in pain.

What mothers mean by this, and what acoustic analysis confirms, is that the cry comes on suddenly and reaches its peak intensity very quickly. We hear that intensity as loudness, a higher pitch, and more noise. In fact, some mothers say it is more like a scream than a cry. One mother said, "He is scream-ing at the top of his lungs."

There is published research on this, our own as well as others', showing that acoustic features such as pitch do change during a colic episode. They don't change for all babies, and not all acoustics change in the same way. But if you are the parent of one of these babies, you don't need any fancy acoustic analysis or research publications to understand what I am saying. But it's nice to have the data, because it supports, confirms, and validates what you're hearing. When a baby has colic, it feels as though she is out of control. This is uncontrollable crying. And she does not want to be doing it. This is not like the hungry cry that says, "Mommy, please feed me," or the teasing cry that means "I want to play." The cry for attention can almost be cute. "Okay, I'll pick you up. You're so demanding," you say to the baby, loving every minute of it. You might even say, "You're such a pain in the ass." But you say it with a smile on your face. But a colic episode is not like that at all.

So what happens when your baby is screaming out of control? You want to help her. She is saying, "Mommy, Daddy, make it stop!" But you can't. And that can make you feel helpless and inadequate as a parent.

The third attribute, physical signs, is actually a group of characteristics that describe changes in the baby's body during a colic episode. (Again, same qualifiers as before: Not all babies have them. Most babies show some of these signs, but not all of them.) The baby pulls his legs up into his chest. He gets doubled over, which is why mothers often say his stomach hurts and he looks and sounds as if he is in pain. His stomach gets hard and his leg and arm muscles get tight. (The technical term for this is *hypertonia*, which means increased tone, or tension, in the muscles.) His face gets red; there may be episodes of breath-holding. His fists clench—sometimes squeezed so tight that you can't open them. It is almost as if the baby is holding on for dear life. The color in the wrists and fingers can get red or white. Sometimes the arms and legs stiffen and stick out straight.

The fourth characteristic is inconsolability. It may sound silly after all this to say that a baby in a colic episode is inconsolable. But the reason we included it is to underline what I said before: You really can't stop this. You may be able to ease it somewhat, reduce some of the crying, perhaps reduce some of the intensity, and make the baby more comfortable. But you won't really be able to stop it. Inconsolability happens when a baby is in an insulated cry state. This means there's a wall between him and you so that you can't really reach him the way you can when his cry state is normal. You need to know, though, that this thing is going to run its course. If you accept that, it will be easier and less frustrating for you—and for the baby.

You can see that by equating colic with excessive crying we run the risk of calling colic "normal" and missing a lot of other cry characteristics that colicky babies have. If it's just about excessive crying, it's easy to conclude that there's nothing wrong with colicky babies. Babies can be excessive criers but be in a normal, not insulated, cry state. These babies do not show any of the true colic characteristics.

The problem we get into here is what clinicians call "caseness," the question of when a problem is a problem. When are the symptoms of a problem severe enough to warrant a diagnosis? If all babies increase their crying during the first few months, when does crying become a clinical concern? When is it a true syndrome? When is it colic?

I have already given you part of the answer. It has to do with how much the baby is crying, along with the additional symptoms—special episodes with sudden onset, changes in the cry, physical signs, and outright inconsolability. But there is still one critical ingredient missing, and it's this: The crying has resulted in some problem either in the infant or in the family. In other words, colic is not just the crying. It's the fact that the crying has caused a problem.

Think about other childhood problems and you'll see what I mean. How do we diagnose a child with hyperactivity? Hyperactivity means the child is very active. But it means more than that. We don't diagnose hyperactivity only on the basis of how active a child is. It is diagnosed because it has come to somebody's attention. The parent complains to the pediatrician, the child care worker complains to the parent, the teacher says the child is disrupting the classroom.

This is where colic belongs. This is why simply using the Rule of Three is like diagnosing hyperactivity strictly on the basis of the child's level of activity. A kid can be very active without having a diagnosis of hyperactivity. A baby can cry excessively without having a cry disorder.

Colic as a diagnosis requires other factors, such as a parent's complaint, a doctor's referral, additional symptoms, or some indication of impairment or dysfunction in the infant's life that is associated with the crying. So let's agree that excessive crying alone is part of normal development at this age—and get real about defining colic.

The way I define colic means thinking about it as a behavioral disorder—and that is why the parallel with hyperactivity works. As with hyperactivity, I use the kind of classification scheme for disorders that we use in psychiatry, the *Diagnostic and Statistical Manual of Mental Disorders*, fourth edition, text revision (DSM-IV-TR). However, we don't really talk about mental disorders in infants, which is why I use the term *behavioral disorder*. The DSM-IV-TR classification system has been so useful that it has been adapted by pediatricians for the diagnosis of childhood mental disorders. It's called DSM-PC. (The PC stands for *primary care*, not *politically correct*, although it is that too.) It was also adapted by the National Center for Clinical Infant Programs, which developed the Diagnostic Classification: 0–3 for disorders of infant mental health. Neither of these classification systems includes colic, because they don't deal with babies this young. But we have applied this approach to colic, and it works well.

In the DSM-IV-TR, a mental disorder requires clinically

significant distress (including distress in the family) or impairment of functioning. So if we regard colic as a behavior disorder, infants with excessive crying that causes clinically significant distress in the family or impairment in the infant would be said to have colic. On the other hand, a baby with excessive crying that causes no significant distress in the family or impairment in the infant would not be said to have colic.

Two criteria need to be met in order to diagnose colic: First, there is a significant complaint of a persistent pattern of crying that is more frequent and more severe than is typical for babies at this age. This can be a disturbance in the amount, frequency, or quality of crying. There may be excessive crying (Rule of Three) as well as symptoms such as sudden onset, high pitch, physical signs, and inconsolability. Second, there is clear evidence of impairment in other areas of function. This could mean that the behavior is affecting the baby's development or other behaviors, the two most common being sleeping or feeding. Or the behavior could be causing stress in the parents, affecting family function and the marital relationship. It could be affecting the parent–infant relationship. There may be attachment or bonding problems. The parents may feel inadequate, suffer loss of self-esteem, and feel ineffective as parents. They may feel angry and disappointed that their baby is acting this way.

I said earlier that you don't have to know the cause of colic to diagnose it. If you use the definition that I just gave you, that's true. But there are a few things that do shed some light

on what causes colic. For example, sometimes the colic is related to another behavioral disorder, such as a sleeping disorder or a feeding disorder. In these cases, whatever is causing
the other disorder results in colic symptoms. Treating the
other disorder can reduce or eliminate the colic. We often see
babies in our clinic who come to us for colic, but we diagnose
the primary problem as a sleep disorder. We treat the sleep disorder—and it helps with the colic. Sometimes something is
going on with the baby medically that results in colic symptoms. This could be GER or an allergy to cow's milk protein.
We treat these conditions—and it helps with the colic.

There is more than one cause of colic. Some of what we
see as colic is related to a greater or lesser degree to other problems in the baby. Some of colic is just the baby's internal system and has nothing to do with other problems—it is internal
baby physiology kicking its heels. The good news about thinking of colic this way is that it points us in different directions
for treatment. If the baby has reflux, for example, you treat
him or her differently than a baby with a sleep disorder or no
other disorder.

There is one more kind of case we see. In this situation,
the conditions for colic are not met. There's no cry disorder
and no impact on child or family, but the mother is having
trouble managing the infant's crying. She may even think or
tell her pediatrician that her baby has colic because for her the
baby's crying is a problem. Just because there is a cry complaint, does that make it colic? I say no. You can't have colic

without a cry complaint, but just having a cry complaint does not make it colic. In this case, we have a relationship problem in which a mom seems to be having trouble with normal infant crying. There's nothing wrong with the infant, but Mom probably needs help managing this aspect of normal development.

There's also the worrisome scenario in which an infant does have the symptoms of colic but it is not recognized as a problem in the family. Just because the family doesn't call it colic doesn't mean that it's not colic and that the family doesn't need help. I wonder how many families fail to recognize that the baby's real problem is colic. They call it something else or they refuse to acknowledge that the baby has a problem at all. In the long term as well as the short term, these babies and their families will suffer unnecessarily. Recognizing colic reminds me of the first time I saw a shark while scuba diving. I was swimming among all these beautiful, multicolored tropical fish and all of sudden there was something in front of me that was out of proportion to everything else swimming around me. Immediate recognition! Colic is out of proportion to regular crying. Just as with a shark, you know it when you see it. And just like a shark, it can chew you up and spit you out.

In chapter 2 we talked about the different kinds of colicky cry patterns that babies have, such as the exploder and the escalator. As you think about how to define and diagnose colic, remember that colic comes in many forms and shapes. There are babies who have colic from day one and there are babies who are angels for the first month and then let you have it. There are babies who have their colicky episode only in the evening and are calm the rest of the time, and there are colicky babies who are never calm or who have their worst episodes at other times of day. Take heart, parents. Don't feel bad if your baby doesn't fit the mold. There are probably as many colic molds as there are colicky babies. The key is to understand what colic is so you can help your baby and help yourself.

Now that you know what colic is and what colic is not, you want to know if it can be prevented. Dr. T. Berry Brazelton, whose books on the Touchpoints Model are my favorite books on parenting, does think that colic can be prevented. Is he right? Well . . . not really.

His approach is based on a wonderful concept that he originated called anticipatory guidance. It means that if you are prepared for something, it is less of a surprise and you are better able to deal with it. In the case of colic, this means that if parents know that it is normal for crying to increase in the first 6 weeks, they can expect it, prepare for it, and be better able to manage it. They will be less likely to define it as a problem and it will be less disruptive to the family.

At some level, this is true. It really does help to know the normal developmental course of crying. Knowledge is prevention and knowing about crying can lessen the impact. But I view this as harm reduction, which is different from prevention. Dr. Brazelton's anticipatory guidance is effective in that it can help reduce the mislabeling of normal crying as colic and help parents manage the increase in crying that is part of normal development. It may even help manage real colic. Knowing that colic is coming from the baby, not from you, helps you to deal with it and helps you to avoid blaming yourself. But it will not prevent the colic.

Nevertheless, I would love to try this harm-reduction approach and see if it helped. If I did I would make sure of two things: First, along with the explanation for normal crying would go a heavy dose of empathy and compassion. Second, I would throw out a safety net and make sure that the mothers understood that their babies might get colic anyway and that if they did, the mothers were not to blame. I would tell the moms that some kids just get it and that if that happens, they should get help. The prevention I would focus on would be to prevent the mothers from feeling alienated, from blaming themselves, and not getting help if their babies did get colic.

Colic is not just in the eye of the beholder. It is not just a mother having a problem with normal crying. Colic is an identifiable cry problem in the infant that is causing some impairment either in the infant or in relationships in the family. Something in the baby is causing a problem for the baby or outside the baby. That's it. End of diagnosis. Beginning of treatment.

CHAPTER SIX

Crybaby Blues:
The Double Whammy of
Depression and Colic

Even though it has been several years since the appearance of news stories about Andrea Yates, I am still haunted by them. She was a Texas mother with depression who drowned her five children, ranging in age from 6 months to 7 years, in the bathtub. The story broke as the nation was becoming more aware of depression in general as a significant mental health problem (her case undoubtedly helped the national awareness) and as we were seeing more and more mothers with depression in our colic clinic. In fact, our recent statistics are that 45 percent of the mothers who come to the colic clinic have significant symptoms of depression. This is scary because having a colicky baby is hard enough. Trying to manage a colicky baby when you are depressed is a double whammy.

I remember a patient who came into the clinic dressed all in black with her 3-week-old baby. She was suffering from depression. She said she was having a hard time finding black baby clothes and asked if we knew where she could get some. She was not joking. It was a sad situation, and her case actually got quite a bit of notoriety for reasons that I discuss later in this chapter.

Depression is more common than we think. Worldwide, the World Heath Organization (WHO) puts the number of people who suffer from depression at 121 million. The WHO predicts that by the year 2020, depression will become the first cause of disease burden in the world. (*Disease burden* means the number of years someone must live with a disease.) Each year in the United States, 12.4 million women experience a depressive disorder, according to the National Institute of Mental Health.

Moreover, women in their childbearing years are at high risk for depression. A recent study from Boston revealed that one-third of twentysomethings succumb to it. Maternal depression that occurs shortly after the birth of a baby, called maternal postpartum depression, occurs in about 20 percent of new mothers. It is probably the most common unrecognized postpartum complication.

The psychiatric definition for maternal postpartum depression is essentially the same as for any major depression. Like any other episode of major depression, the symptoms are dysphoric mood, which means loss of pleasure or interest in usual activities; sleep and appetite changes; cognitive disturbances; loss of energy; and/or recurrent thoughts of death. These symptoms co-occur for at least 2 weeks. This kind of major depression in women is most common between the ages of 25 and 44—the childbearing years. In addition, most episodes of depression persist for about 4 months, which means that postpartum depression and colic will occur at about the same time.

Postpartum depression is severe. It is not just being a little down or a little tired. It impairs the ability to function, to do even normal everyday things like getting out of bed in the morning or taking care of a baby—let alone taking care of a colicky baby. Even when the tasks are normal, everyday chores, the sufferer's affect, mood, and feelings are not normal. It is very hard to avoid communicating these feelings of despair to the baby.

Don't think for a minute, *He's only a baby; he can't tell.* Little babies are nothing but feelings. Crying is all about feelings, and babies have a highly sensitive affective radar system. They know exactly what is going on. In fact, in some ways they know better than adults. That is because babies don't have the cognitive structure and layers of psychological filters to interpret, redirect, or deny feelings that we "sophisticated" adults have. They can sense a depressed mother's hopelessness. They "catch" their mothers' negative emotion and get the message that she doesn't want to be with them. They feel afraid. They feel rejected. They may even feel hostile.

So if you are depressed, you need to understand how seriously postpartum depression impairs your ability to function at a time when being able to function adequately has a whole new meaning because you have a baby to care for. You have a family. A fair amount of research, not with colicky infants but with the ordinary, garden-variety Gerber baby, shows that when mothers are depressed, the quality of their relationship with their baby suffers, the quality of their interaction with their baby suffers, and family relationships are disrupted as well. Some of this research says that when depressed mothers are with their babies, the babies cry more. The babies actually withdraw from the mother and try to avoid interacting with her. How sad. Not only that, these parenting and family relationship problems are related to later problems in these children.

It is not hard to see how this would happen. You don't just become a parent instantly (even though it's automatic when your baby is born). Becoming a parent is a psychological process. There is transition to parenthood that normally brings disruptions that take their toll on parents and families. Even in the best of circumstances, this transition for families is a developmentally challenging time with unrivaled demands and unique stresses.

Remember: It's not a job, it's an adventure. And part of it

is the adventure of understanding your particular infant's personality, his unique style, needs, vulnerabilities, and strengths. So here we are in this vulnerable postpartum period that is so sensitive to disruptions in the formation of the mother–infant relationship and transition to parenthood. This already challenging adventure becomes overwhelming when the mother brings an additional burden of depression to the relationship and the infant brings an additional burden of colic to the relationship.

In our research, we studied mothers with and without depression who brought their infants to our colic clinic. One thing we found was that it was not true that more depressed mothers had more colicky babies. This is important because, as we shall see later, it is easy for depressed mothers to think that they caused their babies' colic. We also found that depressed mothers were more stressed about parenting. They found it more difficult to manage the tasks of parenting; their self-esteem as parents was lower; they felt less effective as parents; and the way the family was functioning was less healthy. None of this should be at all surprising, but it is always nice when research confirms what we know instinctively. It is also important information for the naysayers out there who want to say that colic is a self-limiting, and therefore benign, condition. On the contrary, colic is a catalyst for family problems in families who are already stressed. Of course, the good news is that colic can be an opportunity for treatment that can prevent future problems.

It is important to understand why the double whammy of depression and colic is so problematic. Depression is not just another form of stress (although it is that too). There are some unique things about the combination of colic and depression that make this an especially lethal combination. We have already said that depression makes you tired, and that you need energy to parent even a noncolicky baby. We know that colicky babies are even more demanding. Related to the fatigue of depression is apathy. You may not care as much about being a good mother, about being sensitive to your infant's needs. But in addition to these problems, depression actually changes the way mothers perceive and react to their infant's crying.

Remember our discussions about cry perception and goodness of fit? To have a good fit with your baby, you need to be able to do a reasonable job of perceiving your infant's needs. Depression throws a wrench into that system. It affects your ability to correctly read your infant's signals and cues. It alters and distorts your perceptions and reactions to your baby's crying.

Depression causes you to misperceive the cry. It causes you to overreact so that your perceptions and feelings and reactions are exaggerated. And it can do this in either direction. So in one case, the crying bothers you more, makes you angrier, more hostile, and less tolerant, and you feel less like taking care of the baby. In the other case, denial kicks in and you minimize the crying. You perceive the baby as needing less— even though he needs more. The baby's colic is perceived not as colic but as normal or less than normal crying. Now I'm sure someone is going to say that this denial could be a good thing—that the mother doesn't overreact and is less upset by her baby's crying. But denial is not just the longest river in Egypt. The real issue is whether an infant gets his needs met. The issue is whether parenting is compromised.

It turns out there is research on this too, some done by us and some by other people. We have mothers listen to their infant's cries, and then we give the mothers rating scales so that they can rate how they felt when listening to them. And the studies do show that depression causes these overreactions in how people perceive baby cries. We actually divided our mother–baby pairs into goodness-of-fit groups on the basis of how well the mother perceived her baby's cry. We did a follow-up and found out that when there was a poor fit because of things like maternal depression, the infants had lower scores on standardized tests of mental development and language than when there was a good fit. A good fit—when you are accurately reading your infant's signals and cues—means that you provide better parenting, which makes your baby smarter in the long run.

Now we have to add another layer to the spiraling effect of depression. We have talked about the negative feelings that mothers can have about themselves when they have a colicky baby, the blame, the guilt, the self-doubt. All of these feelings are even more exaggerated when maternal depression and colic combine. Depression already sets you up to feel hopeless.

The additional interpersonal dynamics involved in caring for a colicky baby propel the downward spiral, intensifying any doubts a mother already might have had about being a worthless, inadequate parent. Depression makes it easier for her to believe that the colic is her fault. And of course the entire family suffers.

I know I said it before, but I'll say it again: You are not to blame for your baby's colic. And if you are depressed, you are not to blame for that either. In fact, we know that depression runs in families, so there is a fairly strong genetic component to it. You can't blame yourself for your genes. What you do need to do is understand that you have been dealt not one but two difficult hands. You need to get help. Having depression genes doesn't mean you are doomed. It doesn't mean you can't get help. Genes like these are expressed in environments, and how they are expressed can be modified.

Your genes may mean that you have a predisposition or a tendency toward depression. Here's one example of how this might work. Researchers recently found that people with a certain type of brain chemistry gene were more likely to get depression after stress. The gene makes you more sensitive to stress, so in people with the gene, stress is more apt to trigger an episode of depression. Stress? As in pregnancy? Having a new baby? Having a baby with colic? But having a predisposition to depression does not mean that you have no choice or that you can't do anything about it.

For some women, depression is a lifelong battle. For these

mothers, postpartum depression is like an old friend—or really, an old enemy—returning. Other women have their first experience with depression during pregnancy, while for some, postpartum depression is their first bout.

Most probably depression is caused by more than one thing, including genetics and hormonal changes, especially for women who have not had an episode of major depression before pregnancy or postpartum. But regardless of the cause, there are only two treatment options: drugs (antidepressants) and psychotherapy. In the pre–managed care era, it was actually possible to receive both. You could see a therapist for the famous 50-minute hour and also get antidepressant medication. Now most patients get a med check and a pat on the head—but at least the drugs are getting better all the time.

The most popular antidepressant drugs used for pregnant women and new mothers are of the class called SSRIs (selective serotonin reuptake inhibitors.) Serotonin is a chemical in the brain, a neurotransmitter involved in the transmission of nerve impulses. Serotonin seems to help keep our moods under control by helping with sleep, calming anxiety, and relieving depression. People who are depressed don't make enough serotonin, something the SSRIs seem to reverse. Winning the lottery would probably have a similar effect. At least it would pay for psychotherapy.

Prozac was the first SSRI to gain widespread popularity, and now there are other SSRIs on the market as well. The reason medication is an issue for pregnant women is that these drugs cross the placenta and get to the fetus. For new mothers, these drugs can pass to the baby through breast milk. If we had unequivocal proof that these drugs have no effect on the baby, it would be easier for women to decide about using them. But the jury is still out on this issue. It is probably fair to say that most studies do not find that these drugs cause serious harm to the baby. But I say that with two cautionary notes: One, there has not been a lot of research done on this yet. And two, most studies look at fairly gross outcomes in the infants, such as missing fingers and toes. Some experts think that drugs a mother takes for depression may have more subtle effects on the babies' behavior—but this research is just beginning.

All of this brings me back to the depressed mother dressed in black and looking for black baby clothes. Her baby was very colicky. In the initial interview, she told me that she was breast-feeding and taking Prozac. She had been taking Prozac before she got pregnant, went off during pregnancy, but then went back on after the baby was born. I began to wonder if the Prozac could be causing the baby's colic. I sent some of the mother's breast milk to a drug lab and found out that the concentration of the drug in it was substantially higher than what is even recommended for adults, let alone an 8-pound baby! I asked her if she would be willing to do a little experiment to see if the Prozac was causing the colic. She agreed. We put the baby on formula, and 2 days later, the colic was gone.

Meanwhile, I asked her to use a breast pump and keep collecting her milk. The baby remained free of colic symptoms for several days, but I had to make sure it was eliminating the Prozac that made the difference. The only way to do that was to try to bring the colic back with the breast milk. I felt terrible doing that. How could I induce colic in a patient who had just been through hell and saw it vanish almost overnight? But the mother understood the importance of this and agreed. So she started giving the baby her Prozac-laced breast milk in a bottle. Sure enough, within a few days the colic came back, full blown, just like before. As a last step, just to cinch the experiment, I had a sample of the baby's blood sent to the lab. That was the only way to know for certain if the Prozac was really in the baby, and how much was there. Sure enough, the drug levels were once again very high. Of course we immediately put the baby back on formula, and the colic went away. The mother decided to stop her medication while she was nursing to relieve her baby's colic.

But was *she* relieved? The colic was gone, but she was no longer taking antidepressant medication. Her depression got worse, and she had to stop nursing so she could go back to taking her medication. (By the way, we published this study in a scientific journal and it has been used since to caution mothers about breast-feeding and taking Prozac: "Possible Association Between Fluoxetine Hydrochloride and Colic in an Infant." *Journal of the American Academy of Child and Adolescent Psychiatry*, 1993; Vol. 32, pages 1253–1255.)

For pregnant women and mothers who want to breast-feed, this is a real dilemma. We know that untreated depression can cause hormonal changes in pregnant women, and there is concern that some hormonal changes such as stress hormones can affect the fetus. In one of our studies, we found that untreated maternal depression during pregnancy had an effect on the fetuses' heart rate. But we are not sure that SSRIs are completely safe either, and some pregnant women just hate the idea of taking any kind of drugs while pregnant. Some depressed women benefit from psychotherapy, but others do not, so there is no clear choice.

Postpartum mothers suffering from depression who want to breast-feed have to choose between taking drugs and risking making their baby miserable and not taking the antidepressant and making themselves miserable. Like the mom in our study, many mothers are very reluctant to give up nursing. They see it as critical for developing a good attachment relationship with their baby. For some, it is part of what it means to be a "good mother." Quitting nursing to take medication makes them feel guilty. They think they are depriving their infant, and it makes them feel selfish and self-indulgent. Choosing yourself and your own needs over your baby's? How unmotherly! That mind-set contributes to feelings of inadequacy, as if there is something wrong with them because they have to make this decision.

But if these moms are not taking the drugs and are depressed, what kind of mothers can they be? To a very legitimate extent, taking drugs is really a way of helping their babies as much as they are helping themselves. It enables them to be better mothers, even if they are not nursing.

I have focused on depression because it is important, it is getting more and more attention (as it should), and there is a fair amount known about it. But I don't want to pretend that depression is the only issue out here. What we are really talking about is maternal emotions, maternal psychological states, that can alter parenting. Anxiety and stress are two other examples that come to mind. Many mothers who are depressed are also anxious. Anxiety can make you restless, tired, and irritable. Anxiety and depression can make you feel stressed. These are emotions that change hormones, change brain chemistry, change behavior, change parenting. They can occur alone or in combinations in ways that we really don't understand. But what we can do is put this stuff on the table so we can deal with it.

I don't pretend to have answers for these issues. No one does. These are tough, tough issues, and they need to be acknowledged and discussed. What we should do is to help mothers (with their partners) define these issues, help them articulate their feelings, and help them to find the solution that they are most comfortable with. If you are suffering from depression and the mother of a colicky baby, you must get help. You are not alone. You can beat this. Asking for help, knowing that you need help, is the biggest and most important step you can take for yourself and for your baby.

CHAPTER SEVEN

Don't Cry for Me, Argentina: Lessons from Other Cultures

We have established that all babies cry and that some babies cry more than others do. So crying is universal—but how much babies cry is not. What if I told you that in other cultures, colic is rare and has a very different meaning? That crying is much less common in non-Western, less industrialized, less modern cultures than ours? Does that make you want to take your colicky baby and move to a hut in Bora-Bora? Do you think that if you move to another hemisphere your baby won't get colic? I can't promise that, but what I can promise is that we can learn a lot about ourselves by understanding other cultures—and the benefits of that learning can help us manage our own children's crying. I remember in 1971 walking through a Mayan Indian village in Guatemala called

San Mateo Istatlan. This village is about 12,000 feet above sea level, high up in the mountains. There are no paved roads, no electricity, no McDonald's. You feel as if you have stepped back 2,000 years into history. The people are poor but very proud of their Mayan culture. The silence is stunning and peaceful. It's like the quiet of a virgin forest, but people live here. In the early morning, only two sounds break the silence: roosters crowing and the sound of women making tortillas, their hands gently clapping as they flatten the cornmeal. These sounds echo and reverberate off the mountains.

I have spent lots of time in villages like this in many countries. And what you almost never hear is a baby crying. But on that day in San Mateo, a baby cried. And it was startling. It was riveting. And because it was otherwise so quiet and because we were so high up, the sound of the baby's cry echoed off the surrounding peaks, shattering the silence. People in the village were startled, looked up, and said, "What's wrong?" The crying was an unusual event worthy of notice.

Imagine being in a place where a baby crying is considered an unusual event. We have talked about how baby crying is like an alarm. And that is exactly what happened in San Mateo. It was as if an alarm went off. A siren. *A baby is crying. Why would a baby cry? Something's gone wrong.* This baby was crying because he was in pain.

San Mateo is not unique. Anthropologists have observed that among the indigenous tribes of Tierra del Fuego, babies rarely cried, and then only when they were sick or in pain.

Crying is such a rarity there that adults said that hearing it is the equivalent of having a terrible earache.

In many cultures, *colic* is used to mean the kind of crying that indicates there is something wrong with the baby's digestion. (Remember that the word *colic* comes from *colon*.) Stomach ailments are a real concern in many cultures, especially when poor nutrition is a problem. When a baby cries and there is no real reason for her to be crying—she's fed, she's dry, she's hanging out with Mom—the assumption is that something is wrong with her stomach. Good science aside, if a baby has her legs pulled up so that she is doubled over, her face looks like she is in pain, her cry sounds like she is in pain, and her stomach is hard, it makes sense that it's not her big toe that hurts.

In India, there is almost an obsession with digestion and stomach ailments. At the end of an Indian meal, a tray is passed around with digestive aids such as fennel seeds and betel nuts. Colic is also viewed as a digestive problem, and there are some rituals to prevent it. I was once visiting a Gypsy tribe in India when a baby was receiving a ritual massage. In the beginning, the baby screams as the mother or grandmother slowly kneads his fingers, arms, legs, and so on. It is a slow, tender, intimate process that can take up to an hour. Oils may be used. Toward the end, the baby is held above a fire where incense is sprinkled. The baby inhales the incense and at some point falls into a long, deep, solid sleep. And while the baby sleeps, the mother gets to cook or clean house or listen to music.

As I watched this Indian grandmother undress her baby

(or more accurately unwrap) to get ready for the massage, I noticed what looked like burn marks just below the baby's belly button. There were three or four lines of raised skin, each perhaps a half inch long. They looked like scars from a burn. So, being your standard nosy Western scientist, I asked what those marks were. The grandmother told me they were to ward off colic. The tradition in that tribe was that when a baby is born, you heat up a thin metal rod in the fire and stroke the baby's belly to prevent colic. I guess it worked, because the baby did not have colic. (Of course I'm kidding. Please don't try this!) Most of the studies about how much infants cry have been done in the West. There are studies from the United States, Canada, England, Denmark, and Germany in which parents are asked to fill out cry diaries. But they don't show any consistent pattern. In fact, if you use the Rule of Three, the incidence of colic in these countries would range from 6 to over 30 percent. There seem to be cultural practices that make crying different in different societies. In San Mateo infants are carried all the time, and that reduces crying. There are similar results from Africa, where infants are carried all the time and also cry less. In one survey of over 180 societies, researchers found that infants cried less when they were carried because the mothers were able to sense when their babies were building up to crying episodes. The mothers picked up on their babies' body signals and began soothing before the crying began.

Cultures also differ in how to respond "appropriately" to a crying baby, and what a cry means. In some cultures, a baby's cry is regarded as an ominous sign. In the Celebes, an indigenous people called the Toraja believe that a baby's cry will bring a curse on its parents. The Kurds of Turkey and Iran say that crying is necessary to develop the voice, and so they leave their babies to cry. Taiwanese mothers see crying as a form of infant exercise, and there is even a proverb that says "A child must cry to grow." Clearly, no matter where babies live on the planet, a primary function of parenting is figuring out how to respond to crying.

I have examined babies from all over the world, from India to Hawaii, Latin America, Scandinavia, and Europe, as well as North America. I have also examined babies in many different environments—in hospitals, homes, huts, fields, mountains. I have examined babies in poverty and babies from middle-class families. One thing that is clear is that individual babies, whatever their circumstances, have distinct personalities right from the get-go. Some cry more easily than others do. They seem to have a short fuse or a quick trigger. They are reactive, are easily upset, and cry with little stimulation. Some of these babies are also hard to soothe. When they get "up" (excited, aroused, crying), they stay up, and it is hard to bring them back down. But other reactive babies are easy to soothe. In fact some do what we call self-quieting. You just back off and the baby stops crying by herself (a very popular kind of baby). By the same token, there are babies who are not reactive but still hard to soothe. It seems to take more to get their little cry engines going, but they can still be hard to bring down once they start. I don't think these personality traits are cultural. They just are.

And yet the culture does shape the baby. The "goodness of fit" idea works on the cultural level as well. There are extreme examples of how some cultures handle "mismatches," such as when damaged infants are left to die. But for the most part, the culture sets the norms for what is acceptable behavior and the infant accommodates to them. A culture, then, decides how crying fits in and interprets it accordingly. Anthropological studies have found that in foraging societies; for example, adults in the village react differently to the hunger cry than to the pain cry. If it's a hunger cry, only the mother responds. If it's a pain cry, other people in the village pay attention and respond to the baby. This is because in these societies, the culture defines the mothers' job as feeding, but the entire village is responsible if the baby is in trouble. (Yes, Hillary, it takes a village.)

Can you imagine the foraging society solution happening in Detroit or New York or Charlotte—nonfamily members seeing it as their responsibility to pick up a crying baby that is not theirs? The idea of even paying attention to the type of cry of someone else's baby, let alone acting on it, is foreign to U.S. culture. But think about the sense of isolation and loneliness that so many new mothers feel. They believe they have to shoulder the entire responsibility and burden of parenting, be supermoms. And worse, U.S. culture teaches them that if they need help, they must be inadequate mothers. Yet the evidence from other cultures shows that spreading the job of child rearing among many adults is good for everyone.

From an evolutionary perspective, crying was designed to get Mommy's attention because maybe Baby is hurt or maybe Baby is hungry. This triggers social interaction, the AQ (attachment quotient) goes up, and mother and baby are on the road to a good relationship. To some extent, this is the way it still is in many parts of the world, including San Mateo. Crying is saved for special occasions and therefore has a special meaning.

In modern society, we have changed the way evolution designed the system, and that is why our babies cry more. In most places around the globe, babies are carried or held or in very close proximity to their mothers. So a big part of the communication system between baby and mom is based on noncrying cues such as movement, touch, seeing what the baby is doing, and sensing what the baby needs. Not only is crying unnecessary to summon mom for routine caretaking but it is reserved for emergencies.

Let's go back to San Mateo. Babies there are carried in a sling, sometimes in front, sometimes in back. The mother's sling is called a *juipial*, and it is hand-stitched with very colorful and very beautiful designs. The fibers are natural, the dyes are natural. The *juipial* is basically a poncho. The mother slips it over her head, and it has two vertical slits along the side to make it easier to breast-feed. So when her baby moves or wiggles in some way that the mother understands, she just shifts him around and he starts sucking. No need to cry. The cry circuit has been short-circuited. The baby is never allowed to build up to crying because the mother intervenes way before the baby ever gets that excited. The mother can do this because she is so close and can feel, sense, and see what her baby needs. Crying for routine care is superfluous. At night, the baby sleeps next to Mom and is often so close to the breast that she can nurse while the mom is hardly aware of it. Or, the baby does something and she knows to shift him around and feed—but that something is far short of a cry.

Now let's think about what we do here. We essentially say to babies: "If you want me, call me," or "Cry me." We have altered the original infant–mother communication system to emphasize crying. We put babies in their own rooms and we even use those ridiculous monitors to make sure that we hear every little grunt, peep, and fart. Of course, the real reason we use baby monitors is that we feel so guilty for putting babies in isolation. On some level, we know that little babies were not intended to be put in solitary confinement. But there is more than just guilt involved. We are also worried that the baby will stop breathing. Sudden infant death syndrome (SIDS) is on everybody's mind during the first months, when crying peaks and colic can begin. Our ears are glued to the monitor because we have the fantasy that if the baby is too quiet, she may have stopped breathing. Of course, if the baby were with us, we would not have to worry about this.

Look what else we have done by altering the mother–

infant system to emphasize crying. Babies originally had two separate lines of communication that were distinct and clear. Dial *movement* when you want to communicate "I'm uncomfortable, feed me, change me." Dial *cry* for "Help, emergency, something's wrong." It is much easier for the mother and the baby to communicate when both modes are available. By eliminating the movement channel, we have placed a burden on the cry channel. The baby has to use it to communicate two sets of needs instead of one. Mothers have to adapt and babies have to adapt, which is why things get confused.

But hold off making your airplane reservations for Bora-Bora. Evolution is all about adaptation, as is culture. Our culture has evolved in ways that work for us. We did not change the mother–infant communication system because we are mean and nasty. We changed it because it works for who we are today in the United States and in lots of other places. We don't live in thatched huts. Our child care practices are adapted to the needs and demands of our society. There is give and take, and sometimes there is a cost for living the way we do. Increased baby crying is part of the price we have chosen (consciously or unconsciously) to pay.

This is similar to the conflict parents feel about day care. Of course we feel guilty. Kids were not designed to be put in day care, any more than they were designed to cry every time they need us. But moms have to work, and day care is necessary. It is something we did to ourselves, and we have to accept it as part of the fabric of modern society.

We don't have to change what we are doing with our babies. And we probably couldn't change it if we wanted to, any more than we could suddenly say, "No more day care." Practices evolve because they work; they evolve out of necessity. But by understanding how and why they evolved, we get a better perspective. That takes away some of the sting, some of the guilt. The affective—or emotional—charge of our baby's cry is reduced, and when that happens, we are better able to deal with it, and that makes us better parents. We get less hyped, less anxious, less worried, because we understand why things are the way they are.

CHAPTER EIGHT

Becoming Crylingual: How the Science of Crying Can Help You Understand Your Baby

Now that we have explored some of the social and cultural aspects of crying, let's look at the science of this behavior. This chapter is here for a simple reason. When I understand how something works, I feel more comfortable about it because it is less of a mystery. I think other people feel the same way—and I have seen parents in our clinic relax as they begin to understand how crying works at every level—from vocal cords to parent–child relationships.

Crying is sound, and as parents know, it is anything but

the "sounds of silence." Analyzing cries amounts to analyzing sound. Sounds are composed of invisible waves that vibrate at different frequencies; the science of acoustics breaks apart those sound waves into their component frequencies and tells us what those frequencies are. When you play a C note on a piano, the key makes the hammer hit a string that vibrates and produces the sound we call C. Making that piano string vibrate is like striking a tuning fork. Think of that piano string as a baby's vocal cords. Like strings, they vibrate and produce sound that we hear as cry.

How come all babies' cries don't sound the same? For that matter, how come a C on a piano sounds different than a C on a violin or a saxophone? After all, all C notes are at the same sound frequency. Shouldn't they all sound the same? One difference is that sound from a tuning fork is a simple, or single, sound wave. The sound is vibrating at only one frequency. Frequencies are measured in what used to be called cycles per second and are now called Hertz (Hz).

Most sounds are not composed of single, or sine, waves but of many waves at different frequencies called complex waves. Acoustics takes a sound and dissects it into its component waves and tells us how many waves there are and at which Hertz. Acoustics does for sound what a prism does for light. A prism takes white light, for example, and breaks it down into its components at different frequencies of the color spectrum. The prism tells us that the white light we see is not really white but made up of different colors that when combined look to us like white. Same with sound. Acoustics takes the sound we hear and breaks it down into sounds at different frequencies.

The sounds we hear from musical instruments are not pure sounds; they are complex sounds, even though they might start out as pure sounds. You hit the C note on the piano and the string vibrates, producing the "pure" sound. But then the sound wave bounces around inside the piano. Sound is affected by its surroundings. If another note is hit, it will combine with that note. As the sound resonates throughout the room, it continues to change. That same C played on a violin does not start out in a closed chamber like a piano, so the complex sound is different. With a sax, you vibrate a reed, not a string, and the resonating chamber is a tube. The acoustical environment is what changes the sound and gives it its unique qualities or richness. These are called resonance frequencies or formants, and they refer to how the sound is modified, changed, and filtered by the resonating chamber.

A baby's vocal tract is its resonating chamber. It's like a tube—like the sax or clarinet. Both the throat and the mouth change the sound. The vocal cords vibrate at a particular frequency. The sound leaves the vocal cords and bounces around the throat, upper airway, and mouth, all the time changing, until we hear a single cry composed of many sound waves—a complex sound. With acoustical science, we can make a tape recording of the baby's cry sound and use a computer to do what the prism does—break apart the cry sound that we hear into its component frequencies.

There is one frequency called the fundamental frequency (f0). The fundamental frequency is the basic pitch of the cry, which is actually the number of cycles per second that the vocal cords are vibrating. Most babies' voices have a fundamental frequency of around 300 to 400 Hz, meaning that their vocal cords are vibrating 300 to 400 times per second. Then this sound travels up the airway and produces higher frequencies called formants. There is usually one formant at around 1,200 to 1,400 Hz called F1 and another formant at around 3,200 Hz called F2. F1 and F2 are produced in the upper airway. Then there is F3, which comes from the mouth.

Not all babies have cries at these frequencies, and sometimes the sounds of a baby's cry changes. Think of the vocal cords like strings. How would you make these strings vibrate faster or slower? If you pull on them and make them tighter, they will vibrate faster (higher frequency making a higher pitch). If you relax them and they become more floppy, they will vibrate at a lower frequency (making a lower pitch). So babies who have higher-pitched cries have their vocal cords pulled tighter. The vocal cords are pulled tighter by nerves connected to the brain. Just as you can tense a muscle and it becomes hard and tight by the action of your nerves, a baby can tighten control on the vocal cords and make them vibrate at a higher pitch. We even know the names of the nerves that do this; they are part of the cranial nerves 9 through 12, the nerves that connect the larynx (the voice box where the vocal cords are) to the brain.

The larynx is a muscle. One big difference between how we increase muscle tension and what a baby does is that we can do it voluntarily, while a baby—at least in the beginning—cannot. Sometimes adults tense up involuntarily. And when do adults tense up their muscles in a way that is not voluntary? When we are stressed. We get tight. Sometimes when we are nervous or tense, the pitch of our voice goes up. (The idea of using voice analysis to tell when someone is lying is based on the idea that when people lie, they can't control the stress, and this can be detected in their voice.) So it goes with babies. And so it goes with colic.

When a baby's nervous system is stressed, as in colic, the stress causes tension in the larynx, which causes changes such as a higher-pitched cry. Same deal with the upper airway and formants. This is only the beginning of the complexity. The baby's cries do not occur in a vacuum. Like all sounds, what we hear has a signal component and a noise component. The noise is the junk that is not pure sound. In the lab, we can take the cry and determine what percentage of the sound is signal and what percentage is noise. When the signal-to-noise ratio is low and there is as much noise as signal or more noise than signal, we can hardly hear the frequency parts. We mostly hear noise. Noise can sound like the cry is garbled, raspy, that the sound is breaking up, like when you are listening to your stereo and the music sounds fuzzy, not clean (like some of the music my kids listen to).

One thing that can cause noise in a baby's cry is the force of the sound, and this brings us to the final piece of the acoustical cry puzzle. First, what gets the vocal cords vibrating in the first place? It takes energy and force that comes from the respiratory system. A big push of air from the lungs provides the force to start the vocal cords vibrating. When that airstream from the lungs is strong and steady, the cry has more signal. A strong signal also produces a louder cry. If the signal is too strong for the baby's vocal cords, it overpowers the larynx and you get a cry that is loud and noisy. The muscles go into overdrive. If it is not strong enough, you can get a weak and noisy cry.

The respiratory system also controls other parts of the cry, such as the length of each cry burst. A cry is not just a steady sound. You have a cry burst: "waaaaaaaa." Then the baby stops and takes a breath. Then another "waaaaaaaa" and another breath, and so on, as this cycle repeats. The baby empties his lungs after each cry burst, so he has to take a breath to cry again. How long each cry burst is, how long between cries, and when the baby takes a breath are also driven by the respiratory system.

In chapter 1, we talked about how a pain cry is different from a basic or nonpain cry, on the basis of features such as the length of the first cry burst, breath-holding between cries, loudness, and so on. These features are controlled by the respiratory system, which is in turn controlled by the brain. There are other qualities as well, such as a cry's rhythmic pattern.

Does it have a steady repeating pattern or cadence, or does it seem disorganized? Also, sometimes individual cry bursts are so short that they hardly sound like cries. Sometimes these are called cry attempts or short utterances. They last a half-second or so, and the baby goes, "Uh, uh, uh." These attempts can occur in a baby who is lethargic, has low energy and just can't sustain a good cry, or it can happen at the end of a cry period when the baby is cried out and is just winding down.

To recap the mechanics of cry production: The airstream from the lungs makes vocal cords vibrate, producing sound that resonates up the vocal tract. The sound that we hear as cry is determined by a combination of the force of the airstream; presence of signal versus noise; size, shape, and length of the vocal tract; and the tension of cranial nerves connected to the brain.

Before computers, measuring acoustic cry features was difficult and imprecise. A mechanical device produced pictures like this called sonograms.

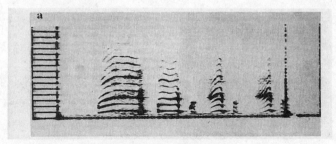

Sound spectrograph of a newborn baby's cry.

This image was made by pens marking pressure-sensitive paper. The marks represented regions of energy where sound was concentrated. The paper is calibrated in Hertz, so when you play a cry, each dark strip means a cry frequency, and the length of each mark is how long the cry sound lasted. The lowest strip is the fundamental frequency, or pitch. These sonograms were somewhat like inkblots—a mix of fact and fantasy. Findings such as very high-pitched cries in babies with medical problems turned out to be true. But other so-called acoustic features that were supposed to be diagnostic turned out to be errors created by the limited technology of the sonogram.

In the digital age, acoustical analysis, like almost everything else, is done by computer and measurement is very precise. Years ago, my colleagues Howie Golub, Mike Corwin, Mark Peucker, and I developed a special computer acoustical analysis system just for infant cries. This turns out to be important because a baby's vocal tract is shaped differently than an adult's vocal tract. We now can create digital pictures like sonograms if we want to visualize the cry. Here is one:

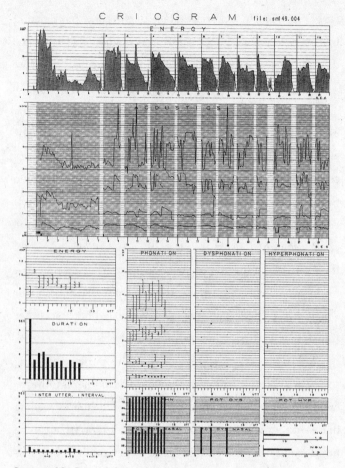

Courtesy of Cry Research, Inc.

Because the information is all digitized, we have the "real numbers" to go along with pictures, and these numbers are what we use in our work. Our cry system does an analysis every 250 milliseconds—one quarter of a second. So four times a second, we get a complete acoustical profile of the baby: fundamental frequency, formants, energy, signal-to-noise ratio, and so on. We do this because vocal cords can change frequencies that fast. Then we average the information to build an overall cry profile.

You can see that there is more to crying than meets the ear. I fully expect that these acoustical analyses will come to be used to help in the differential diagnosis of problems such as colic. Pediatricians could use the information to determine that there is more going on than just how much the baby is crying and confirm what they may suspect is going on from the Colic Symptom Checklist (pages 29–34). Parents could show their baby's cryprints to pediatricians or others who doubt that the baby has colic. And, unlike the Cry Diary (page 28), about which someone can say a mother exaggerated how much her baby is crying, these prints are undeniable proof!

As I sit here typing this, I am on another airplane listening to a baby cry three seats away from me. His mother is trying to entertain him, distract him, by playing with him or feeding him—and it works for reasonable periods of time (that can be measured in more than milliseconds). But I can hear how this baby's cry is changing. Sometimes it is strong and has a clear signal with a steady "burst/pause" pattern of cry-breath-cry-breath. At other times, the pitch goes up. At other times, it sounds almost hoarse and raspy, as if he is gargling. All this from the same baby in the space of a few minutes. Mother and baby are engaged in a cry dance, and it is clear that the mom knows the baby and what his cry means and how to react. She knows when to back off and when to intervene and slow down his buildup. And it is just as clear that the baby knows what he is doing. He is pushing her limits, testing her, yet respecting how far she is willing to let him go. He is backing off at times, changing cry tactics at other times. He jigs. She jags. She jigs. He jags. The difference is that all his jigs and jags are done by changing his cry pattern, whereas she has the full mothering repertoire at her disposal. But guess who's in charge? (If you guessed "mother," go directly to page 1 of this book. Do not pass Go. Do not collect $200.)

The take-home message is that each baby's cry is both unique and not unique. Her cryprint is universal in the sense that it has the same basic elements or features as every other baby's cry. But her cryprint is unique because the way those features are combined is unique to her. No other baby on the planet cries exactly like she does.

That is how and why a mother knows when it is her baby crying. She learns her own baby's cry language. She becomes crylingual. I wish parents could have a cryprint to keep when they take their baby home from the hospital, like the baby's footprint. It might help them appreciate the individuality and uniqueness of their baby, get to know their baby's cry better, and help them become crylingual.

What does it mean to be crylingual? The most straightforward answer is that it means that you understand your baby's cry language, its prosody and syntax. Babies start out with prosody because they are all emotion. Then, as the cognitive layers of the brain come online, they add in syntax. Cry becomes speech and language. That is why becoming crylingual is part of the communication process between you and your baby. You are learning his initial language, and he will eventually learn yours.

Babies, of course, don't cry in a vacuum, so their cries must be interpreted in the context in which they occur. This is not something we think about; most of our initial responses to cry are automatic. We are programmed for many of these automatic responses for basic survival reasons. We jump up (literally or emotionally) when we hear a pain cry long before we can articulate what we are doing. Then we interpret. Your baby cries after he's been sleeping for 3 or 4 hours, and you figure, "Okay, he's up; probably wants to eat." For most mothers and babies, this part of becoming crylingual is relatively straightforward. The dynamic can become more complicated if the baby is a poor communicator. Some babies' cry signals are not as clear as others, and this will show up in the acoustic analysis. The temporal organization or patterning of the cry can be arrhythmic and disorganized. The pitch may change a lot, going up, making you think there is something wrong, but then coming back down quickly so that you think the baby is okay. There can be a lot of noise in the cry. The cry can be very loud or very soft or change a lot between loud and soft. All of these acoustic features make it harder to read the baby's cry signal.

When this happens, the problem parents have is deciding whether the difficulty is really coming from the baby or whether instead, they are somehow misinterpreting the cry. Parents who are more anxious and filled with doubt are of course more likely to think it is them and not the baby. This is why I have stressed that your baby has universal cry features and individual cry features. The *range* of individual cry features is pretty big. Just because your baby doesn't sound like the baby next door doesn't mean there is something wrong with your baby. Babies come into this world wired differently, and some babies take a while to get their act together. Understanding the science, the wiring diagram, and the acoustics of crying helps you become crylingual. It gives you a language, a vocabulary, a way to describe and categorize what you hear. It helps you get to know your baby better, to feel more connected to him. You are speaking his language. You have a language for discussing him with your family and friends. You have a way to keep track of changes. "Gee, have you noticed how much more rhythmic his cry is?" or "He doesn't cry as loud when he is hungry." And if there is a sudden change that worries you, you will have the verbal tools to describe it: "He has these episodes where his cry gets really high pitched, and he didn't used to do this."

Your part of becoming crylingual has to do with how you perceive and react to infant cries. This is called cry perception, and like baby cries, it has universal characteristics and others that are unique to the individual. Not all parents perceive all cries the same. Thinking about your own reactions to your baby's cries will help you to become crylingual.

There is a lot of research on cry perception that has helped establish what is common to all listeners. Researchers, including those I have worked with, such as Dr. Sandy Zeskind and Dr. Zack Boukydis, have asked all kinds of people—parents, nonparents, men and women, students, grandparents, and kids—to listen to tape recordings of baby cries and mark their reactions on a piece of paper using specific categories, such as "How upsetting was this cry to you?" Researchers have also used physiological measures such as heart rate and skin potential to measure how aroused or anxious people get while listening to baby cries. There are certain cries that everyone agrees are very upsetting and aversive. As you might expect, these are clear-cut cases, such as the high-pitched cries of babies who are brain damaged. On the other hand, there are cries of easy-temperament babies that everyone agrees are not upsetting. With these kinds of cries, people are more likely to say, "It makes me want to pick up and hold the baby." These cries are not aversive, and they trigger caretaking.

But apart from these common ways of reacting, we also have individual reactions to baby cries. Some people react more extremely than others, and some people hardly react at all. And while it is easy to get consensus on the high-pitched cry that sounds like fingernails on a blackboard and sends chills down your spine, it is not so easy to get consensus on the less extreme cries that the garden-variety baby has. Two mothers can listen to the same cry of a typical healthy baby and have very different reactions. The same cry may bother one mother and not another. What matters is your reality, what the cry means to you, because that will determine how you react. And if you are aware of these feelings, you will be more crylingual and a better parent. More variables determine how you respond to your baby's cry. People just have different thresholds for what makes them react. Think of how you react to stimulation in general. Are you reactive to sudden sounds? Do some kinds of sounds bother you more than others? Do you have a high or low tolerance for social interaction? The way *you* are wired—how your nervous system reacts to stimulation—has a lot to do with it.

Knowledge and experience with babies makes a difference. If you have had a lot of experience with babies, you know more about what to expect. You will have a model in your head that you can use so that when you hear a new baby cry, you compare it with the model.

If you don't know that much about babies, having people around who do can also help. In one of our studies, first-time mothers and mothers with less support tended to overreact to cries. They were very upset by cries that did not bother other mothers. Teenage mothers, in particular, who had a more immature understanding of babies, also had more extreme reactions to baby cries.

There are also mental health problems that can change how you react to baby cries. Depression, for example, can change a mother's perception of her infant's cry. There are even studies that show that mothers who have abused their infants have extreme reactions to baby cries. For the everyday parent, the important thing to understand is that people can have very different reactions. We react because of who we are, and we should not feel bad if we don't have the same experience as others. But having said that, I also feel that a little introspection can go a long way toward better parenting. If you understand your own individual reactions, when the crying upsets you or what about the crying upsets you, you will be better able to manage your baby. First, there is no need to judge how you feel about your baby's cry. Just accept it. "It really bothers me when he gets into that high-pitched shriek," or "I can take it for about two hours; then I get really pissed." These are legitimate feelings, and they should be acknowledged and not judged. Once you do this, it frees you up. You move on. The feelings do not get in the way. You can see the baby more clearly and get on with the business of parenting. If you feel the need to go deeper and find out why you feel the way you do, seek clinical help—but let yourself off the hook.

Becoming crylingual means giving yourself and your baby permission to be who you are. You learn her language and accept who she is, and she accepts who you are. This is successful parenting.

CHAPTER NINE

From Gadgets to Gripe Water:
Attempts to Treat Colic

How's this for a recipe? Dill oil or dill water, sodium bicarbonate, and 3 to 5 percent alcohol. That's a formula for gripe water, long a popular potion for colic in the United Kingdom. (By the way, gripe water is illegal in the United States. If you fly to England to get some, it will probably be seized by customs officers when you get home.)

Gripe water is one of scores of colic cures that are touted in baby magazines, mothers' support groups, and—especially—on the Internet. Another offering is a vibration unit that attaches to the crib springs and comes with a noise unit to mimic the sound of wind whooshing past a moving car.

Then there are homegrown solutions, such as propping the baby up on a running clothes dryer, running the vacuum cleaner outside his room (or taping the noise of the vacuum cleaner so that you don't completely wear out your carpets), or leaving the shower running while he sleeps. You can spend a bundle on monotonous tapes, CDs of a mother's heartbeat the way it sounded from the womb, white-noise machines, or lull-aby tapes (including a "Jesus Loves Me" edition). You can try swaddling the baby tight (popular in many cultures), carrying her in a sling or a pouch, plunking her in a mechanical swing, warming her tummy with a hot water bottle or heating pad, walking her up and down the stairs, using baby massage. There's nonalcoholic gripe water made with ginger and fennel (Baby's Bliss) and one with peppermint and spearmint and "a barely detectable amount of alcohol." Also touted are aro-matherapy oils, pacifiers, swings—and even cranial massage. There are tight fabric bands for baby's belly, lactase drops, spe-cial bath powders, baby bottles, recommended feeding posi-tion, and exercise routines.

Yes, as any mother of a screaming baby has discovered, whether she searched the Internet, called Grandma, or asked her mothers' group, advice is rampant. The very fact that there are so many gadgets out there, and that parents buy them by the thousands, tells you how desperate parents feel when they have a colicky baby. They'd like to understand what the baby is trying to say. Failing that, they'd like the baby to stop! So they drop their money on everything from gripe water to New Age nonalcoholic teas, stimulating baby seats (nobody wants to say "vibrators"), to special pacifiers. I have a collection of these products on a shelf in my office at the clinic—the Barry Lester Colic Gizmo Museum (admission free). But I don't recommend any of them.

In Europe, parents can buy a device called WhyCry, which interprets infant cries and translates them into English. It reportedly analyzes the frequencies of the cry and its intervals and associates them with an established cry pattern programmed into the unit. After a 20-second period of analysis, it shows the result with a display of one of five simple facial expressions: baby is hungry, bored, tired, stressed, or annoyed. All this for £66—about $114—and it doesn't work.

The problem with colic gadgets is that all of them work once in a while, but none of them work all the time, or even most of the time. In other words, you can always find some cases in which these gadgets do work. And you find plenty of cases in which they don't—probably more than when they do. So, you might ask, what does the research show? Well, there was a study published that analyzed all the results of the gadget studies. Lo and behold, findings showed no evidence that any of these gadgets was effective. (Research on voodoo to get rid of colic is still incomplete.)

The second reason that I am not a gadget fan is that gadgets become just one more opportunity for parents to feel like they failed. And guess what—you don't need this. So a couple tried Gadget X and it worked. They swear by it. "Incredible! We plugged it in, and the colic went away. It's the magic bullet." Then you try it and it's a bust. You went out and spent

$100 for the cure and it doesn't work. All you can do now is blame yourself (again) and say, "It worked for the McGillicuddys, and their baby has worse colic than my baby! But my baby's still screaming. What's wrong with me? Why can't I do anything right?"

The one positive thing about gadgets is that if they do work, go for it! Sometimes I worry that parents' reliance on gadgets could come between mother and baby, becoming a substitute for mother–infant interaction. And that does happen. But in many cases, what the mother gets is a well-deserved break. And the bottom line is this: If you have a screaming kid and there is something that does help, you will use it. It's hard to argue with that.

This caution to be mindful has to do with teaching babies self-regulation. At some point, babies do have to learn to control their level of arousal, to modulate or regulate their behavior. In some ways, you can think of colic as a failure in behavioral regulation. The baby is unable to inhibit his arousal, to stop himself from building up and getting too excited, so he cries. Once he gets going, he can't bring himself back down. His crying escalates until he can't not cry. So he relies on you to handle regulation for him. You become his behavioral regulator.

Behavioral regulation is one of the primary tasks of infancy. We all learned to self-regulate at some point, but like babies, some of us are better at it than others. We all know children and adults who are impulsive or who can't control their behavior. The more you do it for your baby, the harder it is for him to learn to do it for himself. To the extent that gadgets take over and do the regulation for the baby, the baby is not learning what he needs to learn. Probably the most classic example of this, which I have heard from so many mothers, is the famous 2:00 AM car ride. You put the screaming meanie in the car seat, start the engine, enjoy your neighborhood while everybody else is in bed, and just like magic, he goes to sleep. You're thrilled. You can't wait to get him home and upstairs in his crib so you can tuck yourself into bed. You pull the car into the driveway, turn off the engine, and "*Waaaah!*" He's up! You figure *Oh, maybe he wasn't "really" sleeping,* so you do a few more trips around the block and try again. Back in the driveway, turn off the engine, and "*Waaaah!*"

Most parents only need one night of this before they find out it doesn't work. It doesn't work because the baby can't self-regulate. The car is doing it for him. The vibration is his regulator. It is controlling his arousal. He is not. So as soon as you remove the control, he deregulates. Think of it as a braking system (might as well; you're in a car.) The vibration puts the brakes on the baby's arousal. It does the inhibition for the baby. Take away the brake and he gets revved. The control is external when it needs to be internal.

Let me tell you about a case that was a very extreme example of this problem but highlights it beautifully (if unfortunately). The mother brought her baby to the Colic Clinic, and the baby was crying (make that screaming). Mom had the baby on her shoulder. She was walking and patting and jig-gling and rocking the baby. It was all very appropriate; she was trying to do anything she could to calm the baby down. She also looked miserable. Her face was drawn and sad, and she was either very tired or very depressed or very both. I wanted a member of our staff to talk with her and get some basic intake information—and I also saw an opportunity to help. So I said to her, "Why don't you let me hold Sam so we can ask you some questions and you can get a break?" She was startled. She said, "You want to hold him?" And then she said, "Nobody can hold him but me. He won't go to anyone but me."

This turned out to be a very complicated case because the mother was clinically depressed and was locked into an un-healthy, symbiotic relationship with her baby. She really did feel as if they could never be separated. I said, "Why don't you let me try," and she gave me the baby. Later she told me that she couldn't believe that I actually wanted to take this scream-ing baby and that she loved the fact that I used his name—because these two things said to her, "Maybe he's not a monster. He's a real person that someone else would care for."

So I took this kid and kept doing what mom had been doing—walking jiggling, patting, rocking with him high up on my shoulder and screaming in my ear. This kid had one of the worst, high-pitched, irritating cries that I have ever heard in a colicky baby, and it was right in my ear. I was thinking, *I don't know if I can stand this*. And then I felt guilty for thinking about myself and thought about his mother having to deal with this all the time. Then something remarkable happened—and that's why this story is here. Baby Sam went limp on my shoulder. Asleep. He was literally screaming one moment and sleeping on my shoulder the next. There was no modulation of arousal. No behavioral regulation. No gradual transition from cry down to lower levels of arousal. He went from screaming to sleeping in an instant. He was a classic "light-switch baby": on or off. Nothing in the middle. I have seen other cases like this, but this was the most dramatic.

Well, you can imagine how relieved we all were to get some peace and quiet and get on with the interview. I just kept walking and rocking and thanking my lucky stars that the crying had stopped. Then the interview was over and I had to examine the baby. I very gently eased Sam off of my shoulder onto the examination table. And you guessed it: Before he was even on the table, he was screaming again. Just like before. Again, no modulation. The baby light switch was on.

The same principle applies to car-ride simulators that go under the mattress. They may put the baby to sleep, but when they stop, the baby can wake. And—just as important—the baby is not learning to put himself to sleep. Think of crying and sleeping as two sides of the arousal coin. Both are about inhibition, or behavioral regulation. To not cry is to inhibit arousal. To not wake up when you are asleep is to inhibit arousal. To put yourself back to sleep is to inhibit arousal. This, of course, is why so many colicky babies have sleep problems. To add yet another burden—teaching your baby to self-regulate—to the already overwhelmed life of a parent with a colicky baby seems unfair. But part of parenting is teaching. My hope is that instead of seeing this as a burden, you can see it as an opportunity. In the long run, teaching your baby how to regulate her behavior will pay off for both of you, immediately with things like crying and sleeping and later on with temper tantrums. And it will help when she gets to school.

I am reminded of a case in which I was helping a mother in a country on the other side of the world through e-mail, something I don't normally do. But this mom sounded really desperate. It was a classic case of the baby showing all of the symptoms of colic and the mother being told by her health care professional that there was nothing wrong, that she just didn't know how to handle her kid and was just being hysterical. I told her what she could do to help the baby and what she could do to help herself. (Don't e-mail me, please. Just keep reading!) About 6 months later she wrote back to thank me and to let me know that her baby is "an absolutely beautiful girl, she has no problems." Then she said, "except for her sleeping at night. She still wakes up at least two times in the night." This is a case in which the colic was successfully resolved but there was a residual, unresolved regulation problem. A baby at that age who wakes in the night should be able to put herself back to sleep. She should not need to call out for momma. I have mixed feelings about this case; in some sense, I feel as if I failed. I know that had we been able to work with this mother in our clinic instead of through e-mail, her baby would be sleeping better now.

Aside from gadgets, there are other interventions that have been tried for colic—pharmacological, dietary, behavioral, and naturopathic, none of which has been supported by research. Simethicone, sold over the counter as Mylicon drops, is supposed to dissolve gas bubbles and relieve colic! The only downside to simethicone is that it doesn't work— although it is one of those remedies that some parents do swear by, and it certainly doesn't hurt. I suppose we could invoke the "no harm, no foul" rule here.

Perhaps, akin to the placebo effect, these gadgets and treatments sometimes work simply because parents feel that at least they are doing something. You feel so helpless and inadequate when you are unable to quiet your baby. Maybe the drops work because believing that it's not your fault and taking the edge off makes it easier to deal with your baby, and that ease effects change.

Changing the diet is another popular remedy that works some of the time, for reasons that are unclear. Once again, this is something that is relatively easy to do and satisfying because at least you feel as though you are doing something. If you are breast-feeding, you can eliminate foods from your diet that are thought to cause colic. Or you might try a hypoallergenic diet that eliminates foods that babies sometimes are allergic to, such as milk, eggs, wheat, or nut products. There are also foods that may make a baby gassy, such as broccoli, which many breast-feeding mothers eliminate from their diets. (Some mothers just want any excuse to not eat broccoli, colic or not). Coffee, tea, chocolate, and other caffeine products are also eliminated because the caffeine can jazz up the baby.

A word on colic and breast-feeding: As we have seen, crying is part of the developing mother–infant relationship, and to some extent, how much a baby cries and when is determined by how the relationship is set up. Breast-feeding babies tend to feed more often than bottle-fed babies. From a nutritional and health point of view, it has to do with the consistency and staying power of breast milk, and the antibodies passed from mother to baby in it. But anthropologists and evolutionary biologists believe it is much more than that. Breast-feeding keeps mothers and babies in close proximity, so it has survival value. And talk about attachment—you can't be more attached than when you are breast-feeding!

So breast-feeding mothers set up a different kind of relationship with their baby than do bottle-feeding mothers. Breast-feeding babies cry more often to let Mom know that it's chow time. They also get more than sustenance from the breast-feeding. It's comforting and it feels good. So sometimes breast-feeding babies cry because they want to be at the breast even if they are not hungry. You can get into the situation where the baby cries too much because he wants to be at the breast even though he is not hungry. This is not colic, but it can be a problem in the mother–infant relationship. Sometimes you hear that breast-feeding babies are more irritable or colicky than bottle-fed babies are. But I say, *Unfair.* You can't really compare breast- and bottle-fed babies, because their behavior is based on different mother–infant relationship systems. This is yet another reason why the Rule of Three just doesn't work for me; if you just count the hours, you might decide that a breast-feeding baby has colic, when in fact, he is just crying to chow down.

But let's get back to gadgets and other suggested solutions that you might run into on your quest to quiet your baby. There are also "behavioral interventions." Carrying, such as putting babies in a snuggly carrier, does not help with colic. Giving parents intensive training in parent–infant communication skills and reducing stimulation are also techniques that have been tried—but have not been proven effective. Likewise for naturopathic interventions such as herbal teas and sucrose.

An observation I have made but that has never been studied also has to do with stimulation. Some babies are hypersensitive and benefit from less stimulation, while other babies actually quiet with more stimulation. When you have a baby in a carrier, she's getting motion stimulation, but she's also looking around at the environment. She's being stimulated visually and mentally. Now what if the baby likes what she sees? She can't look and cry at the same time. If she wants to look around, she has to keep from crying. She has to control her arousal. She has to regulate her own behavior. She is learning, and you are teaching her (or giving her the opportunity) to develop behavioral regulation.

Some babies can use stimulation to regulate their behavior. I have even seen extreme versions of this with colic, when mothers will take a colicky baby to a shopping mall. Now, you might think this is the last place you would take a colicky baby, and the last thing you want is for your kid to throw a colic fit in the middle of a crowded mall. But some colicky babies are so mesmerized by all the activity and stimulation that it actually keeps them calm. This is using stimulation to self-regulate.

There is a physiological parallel to this. Methylphenidate (Ritalin) is a stimulant. But for children with attention-deficit/hyperactive disorder, it has what is called a paradoxical effect. It calms them down. Malls are not Ritalin for colic. But they do work for some babies. The trick is to know your baby. Throw out the myths, the preconceptions, and all the bad advice and get to know your baby as an individual, as a person. The baby will tell you what he or she likes and dislikes.

One of the hallmarks of successful parenting is the willingness to try new things. Be flexible. Understand that nothing may work—and don't blame yourself and grab the gripe water when that happens. It's not you who has failed. Remember that old saying? If at first you don't succeed, it's probably colic!

CHAPTER TEN

A Colic Case Study:
"I thought I had a handle
on kids"

One of the most insidious things about colic is the way it undercuts parents' sense of competence and robs them of joy. No matter how prepared a new mom and dad may be, no matter how passionately they desired their baby, no matter how strong their support network, the crying can isolate them and make them doubt their ability to parent.

Meet Marian, another mother who sought out our clinic when her son just wouldn't stop crying. When Marian was pregnant with her first child, a baby she and her husband had planned for and awaited with joy, she did what she always does to prepare for something new. She read. An educator, Marian has always done her homework.

"I was prepared," she says. "I have a master's degree in education; I thought I had a handle on kids!" But her son, Zachary, turned every expectation she had on its head.

"I knew it would be difficult," Marian says. "I knew it would be different when it was my own kid. I wanted everything to be as close to perfect as possible for that baby and for our family. I read all the books about preparation and what you should think about in the first year. I had done it all. I highlighted things for my husband to read, too. But I had no idea."

Marian and Bret had no warning that Zachary was going to be anything but perfect. "I had an easy pregnancy. In fact, I loved being pregnant. I enjoyed it, really relished it. I was working; I was starting my business so I was working at home, and I had flexibility and I could keep myself really healthy and exercise and eat well and do everything by the book. I'm not a smoker. I'm not a drinker. I had fruit shakes every day and vegetables every day. I did everything you're supposed to do. So the baby's supposed to come out perfect, you know?"

Zachary arrived 2 weeks early, at 38 weeks. Marian had a fast labor, and her son was born by vaginal delivery.

"He came out and he was fine," Marian recalls. "He was perfect. He gave a major scream when he came out, but that's typical. He came out at 12:01 in the afternoon. From 12:01 until 6 PM, he did not go to sleep. And I was so proud! And the nurses would come in and say, 'I have never seen a baby who stays awake and is so alert.'"

For 2 weeks and 4 days, Zachary was perfect. "At two weeks and four days, we had gone out to a chowder festival. That was the last fun we had for a while. But everything was good. I was nursing and the nursing was fine," Marian says.

Things were about to change. The colic god was lurking in the background.

"That night we went home, and Zachary woke up in the middle of the night," Marian remembers. "He woke up screaming. And we said, 'What's going on here?' And we did everything you're supposed to do: Does he need a poopy change, does he need a pee-pee change, does he need to be nursed, does he need to be burped, does he need to be cuddled? We did all those steps the books say, and nothing was working."

Marian pauses and sighs, picturing those early days.

"I kept trying to fix it. I can't recall how long the first episode of crying was, but it was up there. It was a good amount of hours. My husband and I were passing the baby back and forth. We tried putting him in the little bouncer seat; we tried carrying him around. We thought he was really, really sick—but he had no temperature."

Marian and Bret took their son to the doctor. He said, "'Oh, he could have an upset stomach,' which wasn't much help."

Zachary's crying continued the next day. His parents saw a

second doctor, who said, "Oh, your son probably has colic. It's not a big deal. He'll grow out of it."

Back home, Zachary kept crying.

"I went to the doctor again," Marian says. "I said, 'This is *not* okay. I need to be able to do something. Can you give me literature? Can you steer me in some direction?' And his response, again, was 'It will go away at some point.'

"I was thinking, *They're thinking this is a high-strung, neurotic mom, and that's why her baby is the way he is.* There are a lot of things in the literature that make it sound like colic is your fault."

Marian's support network, usually helpful and responsive, didn't seem to get it. "My mother-in-law, who's really good and really supportive, would say things like 'You know, babies cry. You just need to hold the baby.' And different friends would give that same advice: 'You know, babies cry, and I know it's really hard because it's your baby. You are just going to have to get through it.' I would sit there thinking, *This isn't just crying; this is screaming. This baby is really unhappy. This baby is inconsolable.*"

The relentless crying and her family and friends' lack of understanding made Marian feel terribly alone. "I felt like I was in a little bubble. And it didn't help that my sister had had her first son twelve days before mine. We live near each other. And her son was this really placid, really good baby. As much as it was great because my sister was so supportive of me, I was seeing a child as opposite to my son as a child could be. And I was questioning myself, wondering if because my sister is so much more laid back than I am, I was somehow doing this to my son." Such feelings are common among colic moms.

Other people's innocent inquiries about your baby can add to the strain. "People would say to me, 'How's your son doing?' and I would say, 'Fine, fine. I didn't realize until after about six months that being a mom had turned out opposite to everything I had expected. I had thought I would seek friendships with new moms. But I didn't go to moms' groups. I didn't make those connections, which is so unlike me."

Marian says she had been ready to leap into the community of new moms. "I had a list, I was ready. But I didn't know when he was going to cry; I didn't know when he was going to scream. I couldn't go because I couldn't explain it. I knew that they would walk away and not understand."

The isolation weighed on her.

"I remember one day being upstairs—my son's gorgeous—and looking at this beautiful baby. He's screaming and crying, and my husband had gone to work, and I'm so sleep-deprived and discouraged. All of a sudden, the tears just started to come. I sat there on a chair saying, 'Zachary, just tell me what you want. I will give you anything.'"

Marian sought help through the Internet and found a chat room used by other "colic moms." "I remember sitting downstairs in my office and reading the comments, crying, and thinking, *Oh, my God. Other moms are saying, 'You know I wanted this baby so bad and now I almost want to give it back!'*"

Marian began to reach out a bit more, talking to other moms on the phone. "If you say, 'My baby's colicky,' you get a wide variety of reactions," she says. "But right away you recognize the moms who mean it, who know what you're talking about. I don't mean the moms whose babies fuss at dinnertime. That's not colic. I had a client from my business who shared a lot of information on the phone. She said, 'I know what you are going through. My son had colic. And I remember the only way my husband and I could breathe for four seconds—we lived in an apartment—was we would stroll him outside and put him by the steps and close the door and he would cry and we would eat dinner.' She said, 'No matter what, get someone to watch your child for thirty minutes and go for a walk.'"

Good advice. But Marian found herself unable to heed it until after she had taken Zachary to the Colic Clinic and the family's treatment had begun.

Our clinic uses a multidisciplinary approach, with both a pediatric and mental health component to our services. This approach recognizes that while colic is a problem in the baby, it also affects the family as a whole. When he was first examined at the Colic Clinic, Zachary was 4 weeks old—and was spending up to 10 hours a day crying, typically between 5:00 and 10:00 AM and then again from 5:00 to 10:00 PM. Marian and Bret had tried everything they could think of to soothe him, and nothing was working. "A huge thing that the Colic Clinic did was ask me to fill out charts. Now, the charts are frustrating because you have to take three days in fifteen-minute cycles. It's a huge commitment. But you have to do it. It allows you to validate that this baby really is crying twelve hours in a day. That's not normal; that's not typical. When you see it on the chart, you stop questioning yourself. But it also gives you a chance to see that the crying swings up and swings down. It helps you see that it is going to end."

Marian and her husband also attended a colic parents' group. "Being with a group of people who have been experiencing this day in and day out can validate you. It helped my husband and me because our styles are so different—he would be like, 'It's okay,' and I would say, 'It's not okay.' Going to the clinic meant we could hear each other better. He could hear that I wasn't just a whacked-out first-time mom."

We told Marian to carve out at least 30 minutes of "mom time" daily to read a book, take a nap, or go for a walk. Two weeks later, by Zachary's second visit, his crying jags had shortened. His mom had found that she could soothe him by quietly holding him. He was going to bed earlier, and he was sleeping in his own crib, not Mom and Dad's bed. But he was still having trouble sleeping during the day. By 8 weeks, he was more comfortable, having started a trial of Zantac for his reflux. Five weeks later, things were much better. Zachary was crying less than an hour a day, was able to self-soothe at night, and had started taking naps during the day. Three weeks later, he and his family came to see us, and his parents reported that they had managed a short camping trip to Maine with the baby.

When Zachary was 16 weeks old, he and his mom and dad

finished their sessions at the clinic. "Congratulations! You have graduated," the last communication from our staff said. "You and Bret and Zachary have accomplished a lot. Zachary continues to thrive. He has a regular bedtime preceded by a soothing routine that helps him transition to sleep on his own. Developmentally, he is cooing, smiling, and very interested in his surroundings and likes to stand. He is literally a happy camper, as your recent adventure to Maine has demonstrated!" We advised them, "Continue to have adventures together, both as a family and as a couple."

Zachary is 5 now, an active, sunny boy. But the memories of his colic days linger. "Later, you chuckle about things that you did," Marian says. "The white noise from the TV, driving along a bumpy, under-construction highway at two AM, putting him on top of the dryer. I have a picture of Zachary in the laundry basket on top of the dryer, and he's lying on top of the laundry with a pacifier in his mouth, asleep. Bret and I just stood right there. The baby slept for maybe seven minutes. I am not kidding. We would do three minutes vacuum, seven minutes dryer."

In spite of the memories of their struggle, Marian and Bret decided to have another baby. As with Zachary, the pregnancy and birth went well. "After I had Amy, I was holding my breath until we passed five weeks," says Marian. But her second child was not colicky.

During our interview, the two children woke from their naps and trundled into the living room to see what was going on. Zachary had his arm protectively around his little sister's shoulder. Seeing them, Marian said, "Now, Zachary is truly one of the happiest children alive. If Zachary cries, you know something has happened. He's the warmest, most empathic. He's so giving, so loving. But if you had told me that in that first four months, I would have said, 'Let me have that in writing.' When he was tiny, he was just so serious and so sad."

CHAPTER ELEVEN

Dads Need Help, Too: Colic and the Family

Even though it may not be politically correct to say so, mothers are the ones who bear the brunt of colic. Even so, dads do have a huge role to play. Let's look at what colic does to them. Most dads, whether they acknowledge it or not, assume that Mom is in charge of taking care of the baby. That is not to say that dads don't help but that the executive function, the decision making, and primary responsibility for the baby is usually the mother's. She's the one who keeps track of which "kid things" need to get done and who should do them. In this way, Dad is already one step removed from the baby's care. I know it's not this way for all families, and if yours is not this way, bear with me. I am talking about the majority of families.

Many dads do not consider themselves baby experts. In

fact, some dads feel very estranged from little babies. They feel like they don't understand them and can't relate to them. Some dads are even afraid of babies. They can't wait until the baby can talk. Once babies talk, many dads feel they can finally relate. I hope the dads who feel this way will feel more connected to their baby after learning from this book that babies do have a language. When dads become crylingual, they will be better able to relate to their babies.

The fact is, it's very tough for dads when something goes wrong. They get confused and have mixed emotions, especially when it's something like colic that is poorly defined and controversial in terms of whether it's normal or not. As ironic as it sounds, there is something comforting about hearing that a child has a "real" disease. You can put a label on it. You have a diagnosis. At least you know, and there's no ambiguity. You know that it is not your fault.

But colic is trouble for a dad because it can raise doubts— doubts about his wife, doubts about her ability as a mother, as a parent, as the person in charge of the care of *his* child. Dad may not even be aware that he's blaming Mom for the baby's colic or may not be able to verbalize that he feels this way, but it comes out in his interactions with his mate. He may not be supportive. He may second-guess, criticize, question her management of the colic, and undermine her—making her feel even more inadequate and incompetent and reinforcing her feelings and fears that she is a bad mother. Dad doesn't do this on purpose. But he is confused and ambivalent. He wants to help but doesn't know how. He doesn't want to interfere or take over. He feels helpless and frustrated. Dad feels just as strong an urge as Mom does to help the baby, but from his backseat position, he may wonder, *Do I have the right to say anything?* And of course all of this is magnified 1,000 times if the pediatrician or his mother-in-law or mother or the mom's sister or her friend or their neighbor says, "There's nothing wrong. It's just normal colic." Or worse, "You're _____ing him too much."

The worst fill-in-the-blank—and probably the most common—is "You're spoiling him too much." We hear that so often. Moms are told they're causing the colic by picking the baby up every time he cries, by carrying him, by paying too much attention to him. Attention, mothers and fathers and caregivers of all ages: You will not spoil babies by picking them up! It's good for them. There's even research that found that when mothers picked up crying babies, mother and baby had better attachments later on—and the babies cried less.

Of course, dads are also affected by crying. And they are affected personally. It gets to them whether they respond with guilt, anger, frustration, or withdrawal or are supportive and calm in the face of the crisis. Cry perception studies have been done with dads, and they show the same emotions as mothers. Just because the stereotypical dad is not expressive or demonstrative does not mean that he does not have feelings. Even if dads don't show it, they feel it. They feel bad for the baby and want to help. They also find the cry upsetting and can experience negative emotions, such as anger, toward the baby. They can feel disappointed, and dads also need to understand that these feelings are normal. It is okay to have these feelings about your baby. But it's difficult for Dad because he's not in charge. That's a tough place to be. And it's even tougher if he feels as if he doesn't understand babies very well. If you're used to babies, you know at some level that crying comes with the territory. But if babies are new creatures to you, you may not be prepared for normal crying, let alone colic. You may think, *This is not what I bargained for.*

Dad is also in a bind because he doesn't want to share with Mom how he feels about what the crying is doing to him and how it makes him feel about the baby. A dad often feels that he needs to be the rock, the stabilizer, the go-to guy whom Mom can lean on. He may worry that talking about how he feels about the baby makes him look weak and reveals a crack in the rock. He may feel embarrassed and confused about his feelings about the baby's crying—just as Mom does—and not be sure how to handle his conflicting emotions: *I love this kid and I hate this kid at the same time.*

It's very difficult. And it's not something that comes up as we prepare for parenthood. Even the thought of having negative emotions toward our baby is not something that we are ready to face. Dads may not want to admit that they feel anger or hostility or disappointment toward their babies. They may not want to admit those feelings to themselves, let alone to their wives! I think many dads (and moms too) are actually shocked and overcome by these feelings because they are so unexpected.

As I said earlier, one of the reasons that colic can be so difficult is the shocking way it comes out of the blue, potentially
derailing the parent–baby relationship. But that's just the baby
part. Many dads and moms are also shocked by their own feelings and reactions. Their feelings, just like the baby's crying,
are unexpected. Parents can be overcome by their own reactions and not know how to deal with them, which can get in
the way and even further derail their relationship with the
baby. Now, maybe Mom is comfortable talking about this
stuff—but Dad often is not.

Dad can pay a price for keeping these feelings to himself.
He may feel it's not his place to share the feelings because he
doesn't want to add another burden, another demand, to his
wife's problems with the baby. So he may choose to keep the
feelings bottled up inside and pretend that he can handle it. It's
Macho Baby Dad! When we talk about conflicting feelings,
what happens if Dad does have doubts about how Mom is handling the crying? What if he thinks he can do better? You can
get into a situation in which Mom and Dad are competing with
each other over how to handle the crying. Needless to say, they
can't work together when they're working against each other.
Competition over the baby is divisive not only to the marriage
but also to the parents' relationship with the baby. The baby
will be getting mixed messages, too. And yes, babies can tell.
And yes, they can learn to manipulate the situation and play
Mom and Dad off each other. This is the kind of classic triangular relationship behavior that we usually think of in older

children, adolescents, and adults. But babies can do it, too. Family dynamics can be altered when this happens. I have often heard dads say, "He only stops crying when his mother holds him." When that happens, Dad feels he has no role.

Moms and dads have different ways of handling, holding, and soothing the baby. And dads often have different ways of being with the baby and playing with the baby. Research has shown that dads do more bouncing and "rough" play. They are more likely to poke and prod, to be more physical. This means two things: First, Dad has a different relationship with the baby than Mom does. Second, babies know this. Babies develop different expectations for dads than they do for moms. When Dad comes over to pick the baby up, different lightbulbs go off in the baby's head than when Mom comes over, making the reciprocal process of the parent shaping the child and the child shaping the parent completely different. That's how babies are able to "manipulate" dads differently than they do moms. When Dad picks up a crying baby, the baby is expecting something different than when Mom shows up. And if Dad doesn't do what Dad is supposed to do, the crying might intensify. What's the baby saying? "Hey, Dad—do it the way we negotiated." If it is only Mom who soothes the savage beast but Dad tries to lend a hand, the baby might reject Dad all together. The baby is saying, "That ain't the deal. That's Mom's job."

Dad has got a lot on his plate here. He's feeling, *My job is to support my wife and make things as easy for her as I can, to help her get through this crisis.* That's his bottom line. But then he also has to juggle his own feelings about what the baby's crying is doing to him, how he feels about the baby, his worries about his relationship with the baby, and his disappointment in the baby. And then there's his relationship to his wife (aka partner). He has to deal with his feelings about his wife as a mother (*Is she doing the right thing? Is she spoiling the baby?*), and he has to deal with his feelings about his wife as a wife. As a nonmother. As his lover, his friend, and his partner.

What can happen to the marriage? Well, the marital relationship also gets whacked by colic. And what do you suppose happens to Dad when he feels that the baby's crying is compromising his relationship with his wife? More mixed emotions. More negative feelings. Dad now resents the baby for what the baby is doing to his relationship with his wife. This baby is wrecking his marriage! Dad has these negative feelings piled on top of the other sets of mixed emotions.

Dad wears many hats. He's father to the baby, support to Mother, husband to wife. And he has his own feelings to deal with around each of these issues. And, by the way, he may also be the primary breadwinner, so let's not forget his full-time job of bringing home the bacon. He has to do the father-support-husband thing after work hours. So where does leisure time come in? What about hobbies and fun? Are we having fun yet?

How easy it is for fathers to forget that we also have ourselves to take care of. We have our own needs, that part of us that is not father- or husband- or job-related. When that part gets squashed, denied, buried, and put on the back burner, it also cries out. The little "me" inside feels resentment. We are more than the sum of our parts, but when a part is missing, the whole is diminished. As I said for moms, if you don't take care of yourself, you aren't going to do a very good job taking care of your family. You can't manage your multiple roles very well if your insides are hollow.

I think that it is the imbalance between meeting internal needs and external demands that leads to problems more than anything else. Superdad-Superman is just as dangerous as Supermom. (You never saw Lois Lane with kids, did you?) It undermines families and wrecks marriages. You can't give everything up for the sake of the family. You have to preserve who you are apart from the family. You are still you, and you need to stay in touch with your inner self—even if you do have a colicky baby! You need to feel good about who you are. That will give you the strength to be a good father and good husband. It's Viagra for the ego.

The balance part is critical. I am not giving out a hall pass for Dad to go out and drink with his buddies. It is not as much about doing things as it is about feelings and coming to grips with who you are. The balance I'm talking about is internal. It's about being somewhat introspective and taking the time to figure out what is going on with you. Inside. Then act.

The mother–baby–father relationship is a three-way relationship. A three-way family system. The system has its parts, and the parts interact and affect each other. Mom is the lynchpin that holds the system together. Dad is the bracket. Baby is, of course, the centerpiece around which the system revolves. Without the bracket, the system has no support. All parts of the system have to work for the system to work.

This three-way system is a triangular relationship, and you know what can happen in triangular relationships. One partner is often left out, isolated, ignored, or rejected. Well, if Mom and the baby are the centerpiece and everything revolves around the baby, guess who gets left out in the cold? Dad. Not really left out, but if the mother–infant relationship is priority #1, the other two sides of the triangle—the mother–father relationship and the father–infant relationship—vie to be priority #2 and priority #3. What happens will depend on how the family works it out. As I've said, relationships aren't developed, they're negotiated. Now we have a third party at the negotiating table. Dad says, "I want my share, too." And this is not a static system. It is dynamic. It will change. A crisis like colic can cause a change in the system. It can force the family to shift priorities to take care of, the immediate problem. When the problem is taken care of the family can readjust.

A family comes out differently after a crisis. It has morphed. Now the family has to reinvent itself and figure out what was learned from this experience. How do its members want to be in this next phase until something else comes along to force a change? Maybe what comes along is another external event. Fast-forward 9 months. Now the baby is showing stranger anxiety and clinging to Mom so much that Dad is going nuts. And Dad is feeling, *Hey, what is this? We went through a few months of hell with colic when the kid screamed and my wife had to carry him all the time. I thought that was over. Now he's nine months old and here we go again. He wants to be held all the time! Again.* Or maybe what forces a change is an internal event. Mom or Dad says, "Time out. This is not working for me. We need to change the system. My needs are not getting met." In other words, someone asks to renegotiate the triangle.

Healthy families actually have lots of triangles that together function as a system that accommodates changing situations. Each family is unique and has to develop a system that takes into account the individuality of the baby (the baby's personality) and the individuality, the personality, and the needs of both parents. It helps to think of relationship triangles as models or templates the family has negotiated for different situations that come up in the course of normal parenting. There might be a template for how to deal with the baby's crying, for example, or a template for "going to visit Grandma," among others. Depending on the situation, the triangle may be constructed differently, with roles changing accordingly.

On some level, this is what parenting is all about—trying to negotiate templates that can accommodate to the immediate situation and that are flexible and can adapt to the changing needs of the *three* members of the triangle. It also means remembering that templates have two components: There is the relationship component (our feelings and how we treat each other) and the action component (who does what). If Dad is the most loving and supportive and caring guy in the world but Mom still does all the work, Dad ain't doin' his job. Be loving, but also get up for the 4:00 AM feeding. By the same token, if Dad is Mr. Big Helper and feeds and changes the baby (*even #2!* Come on, guys. I know how some of you brag about changing the baby's diaper, but you do only the pee-pee) but his affect—his expressiveness—is off, that's just as bad. One of the problems that families can have is that they don't change roles or have enough different templates.

The way you handle your crying baby at home might not work in the grocery store or at a party or at Grandma's. Again, it's not just about the baby. It's about the three relationships in the triangle. So maybe at home, the baby cries and the family dynamics are set up so that Mom goes over and picks him up. But let's say you're with Mom's boss and the baby starts to cry. Then you might have a template that triggers Dad to pick up the baby or take the baby from Mom so that she can be more effective with her boss. Sometimes what happens with crying is that family members get stuck. They find a template that works in one situation and they stick to it. They assume that because it works at home it should work everywhere, or that because it worked a few times it should work all the time. What they forget is that even if the baby's crying is a constant, the parents are different people in different situations.

The need to negotiate and change applies to families with normally crying babies, but colic tends to magnify things. Crying is a stressor, and people (parents included) act differently under stress. Maybe one of the reasons that the colic god decided to wait until babies are 4 to 6 weeks old for them to have colic was to give parents a chance to negotiate cry templates around normal crying before hitting them with colic. This makes me really feel sorry for families who have a colicky baby right from the start. We don't see this too often, but it does happen, and those parents don't have a chance to get prepared.

Triangular relationships and shifting parenting templates become even more complicated if there are other children or household members. When parents have to divide their time between the new crying baby and the older child, resentment can easily build. If Mom has to spend lots of time carrying and soothing the new baby, that's less time she can spend with her other children. They may be put off by the baby's incessant crying and even come to dislike their new sib. I have even seen cases in which the older child will develop symptoms—behavior problems—in reaction to the new baby's crying. We had one case in which a 3-year-old who had no sleeping problems and was toilet trained completely regressed when the new baby in the family developed colic. The 3-year-old started wetting his bed, waking up in the middle of the night, crying, and wanting to sleep with Mom and Dad.

The stress of a crying baby impacts virtually all areas of family life. You don't want to take the baby out for fear of her having an "episode"—so you stay home. You become isolated. You stop seeing your friends and family—so your social life and social network is compromised. You may not want to have friends and family visit. You are embarrassed.

Social support is not always as straightforward as we might like. And sometimes family members are so desperate for relief that they take the bad to get the good. You want support, but it may come with baggage, mixed messages, left-handed compliments, or sarcasm. Of course, grandparents are often life-savers and life enhancers, not criticizers and undercutters. Reactions to crying are not going to be as severe as reactions to colic. But if you understand colic as a crisis and severe stressor, it makes sense that some parents choose to withdraw. Conventional wisdom might suggest that when people are in trouble, they need and want help. And some people do react that way. But one of the findings that came out of the social-support research was that in times of crisis with a baby, many family members do not want help. They withdraw. They hunker down, pull in the reins, and build a protective wall. It's the "circle the wagons" idea: Conserve family resources and turn inward. It takes energy to deal with the outside world. Sometimes the psychological cost of getting help is too high. As professionals, we need to respect parents' rights to feel this way, even if we wish it were otherwise.

So far we've been talking about families with a mom (the lynchpin) and a dad (the bracket). What happens when there is no bracket? We know that crying and colic are stressful in the intact nuclear family. What if there is no nuclear family to circle the wagons? Obviously, many single moms handle colic on their own, particularly if they have friends and family they can turn to. But these moms need to know that help is available if they want it. We professionals need to find better ways to reach out to the community and let these moms know that they are not alone. We need to convey to them that we know how serious a problem crying and colic can be, that we know what it does to them and their baby, and that we are ready to help.

Let's think about crying and colic with the concept of differentiated parenting. The concept of differentiation is not new. It has been popularized in regard to adult relationships, particular marital relationships, especially and most effectively by David Schnarch. The essence of the idea is that you need to maintain yourself in the context of a relationship. In a sense it is the opposite of symbiosis. It is preserving your individuality and making sure that your needs are met and are as legitimate as your partner's. Differentiation is similar in the parent–baby relationship—but it's communicated differently. You can say to your wife, "I know we haven't seen each other much lately, and I do want to be with you, but right now I really need some time by myself and then we'll connect." But you can't say that to your crying baby. Nonetheless, the concept is applicable.

Differentiated parenting has two components, the intrapersonal part (how you deal with yourself) and the interpersonal part (how you deal with others). The intrapersonal part within yourself is where you do the psychological work needed to keep your individuality and your personal integrity intact and in the foreground. You do this to prevent yourself from losing yourself. But that is not all you are. Keep track of the parts of you that are not family, the wants and needs and cares and the feelings that have nothing to do with being a husband and father. They are just as much a part of you as the husband-father-family you. Even if you don't act on your needs, know what they are and know that you are choosing not to act on them. If you live blindly, giving up needs unaware, not only will you lose yourself but you will also build anger and resentment. You will feel as if you don't have control. You will feel like a victim who is being buried and destroyed by parenthood. If you consciously put your needs aside, you will feel more in control and able to give to your family in a way that is unencumbered (no strings). The only true gift is a gift without strings, and that is what you want to do as a dad or mom for your family. Hold on to yourself and you won't be a victim.

This idea of maintaining self should not be confused with being selfish. It does not mean, "I got to be me and the heck with Mom and the baby." The ability to maintain your sense of self in a relationship benefits everyone. It lets you be more attentive and adaptive to your spouse and baby because you're not demanding that the "other" support you (your sense of self). Differentiation includes regulating your own anxiety—soothing your own hurts and insecurities, rather than making others soothe you. People who have no self are the most selfish people in the world. Differentiation enables you to put your partner's needs on par with your own—and both your partner and the baby will benefit.

Because this is Dad's chapter, the examples in it are dads,

but everything I say goes for moms, too. So, dads, the interpersonal side of "differentiated parenting" involves how you relate to your wife around your needs, and how you relate to your baby. You need to let your wife know what your needs are and when your needs are not being met. You can't not say what you feel because you are afraid of overburdening her. She has to be able to deal with your issues. That is part of her marriage contract. Just because you have kids doesn't mean that you ignore each other. You have to put your stuff out there. She has to accept it. She might not like it. She might not feel that she can do anything about it. You might fight. But do it anyway. And you, Dad, have to understand that saying is not the same as getting it. Just because you put it on the table doesn't mean you have any rights to get what you want. It just means that you have the opportunity to articulate your feelings. Your wife will probably appreciate your being forthcoming even if she doesn't like what you have to say. Together, you may be able to find alternatives or look for solutions, or you may decide that right now in this time and place there is no solution. At least you are going into parenthood with your head held high, in control, and with your dignity and integrity intact.

So what kinds of issues are we talking about here? Anything and everything. It might be a night out with boys—or something more delicate, such as you want sex and she isn't ready. She goes to her 6-week postpartum gynecological checkup and gets the green light for a little fun in the sun. She is not sure that she is up for it. She is still feeling fat, stretched, and out of shape.

She is breast-feeding and worries that it will interfere with sex. She is tired, and all she can really think about is the baby. But she knows you are getting horny. You've been making moves at night. She doesn't want to disappoint you. She doesn't want you to have an affair. Does she tell you that she saw her doc and the runway is clear? You know that your wife saw her doctor. If she doesn't tell you what the doc said, do you ask?

And what if you don't want your wife to keep breast-feeding because you like her breasts during sex and to you, the milk is a real turnoff? Is this another joke by the colic god—that at 6 weeks, crying peaks and the baby gets colic just as your wife is cleared for sex? And there's another conflict: Your wife is in love with the baby. She feels as if she is cheating on you. She may think, *This can't be. I love my husband and I love my baby, so why do I feel guilty?* You feel it, too. You feel as if your wife loves the baby more than she loves you. Then, of course, you feel ridiculous—competing for your wife's love with a 1-month-old baby.

What's this all about? Well, it's about reality, because that's exactly what is happening. Dads need to know that their feelings are not ridiculous. So, Dad, if you want to get through this and keep your sanity and keep a healthy relationship, you have to do two things: (1) keep your sense of humor and have a laugh over the irony of the colic god's taking your wife away just when you thought you were getting her back and (2) make an appointment for a marital table talk. Get someone else to take care of the kid so that the two of you can have some time alone.

Tell her you love her. You miss her. You find her sexy. You want her. And be prepared in case she says no. And then tell her you love her and schedule another table talk.

One of my favorite images of a father in touch with his needs is the guy who is bicycling and pulling the baby behind him in what looks like some kind of Roman chariot. Every time I see something like that I think, *Yes! You go for it, Dad.* Because here is a guy who simply says, "Just because I'm taking care of the baby doesn't mean I can't go biking." Dads also have to give themselves permission to do things their own way. Becoming a father is not just becoming a mother replacement. It means giving your child a different, complementary relationship.

Dads have to define fatherhood for themselves. It starts from day 1, and early crying or colic may be Dad's first test, the first time he has to rely on his own resources as a parent and figure out what to do. You get to define your own identity as a dad as you cope with and manage your baby's crying. This becomes part of who you are. It builds your ego as a dad. And like those discussions with your wife we just talked about, it is proactive. You are doing. You are in control. You are building yourself as you build your relationship with your baby. You are solidifying your *self*—and that's becoming a differentiated dad.

CHAPTER TWELVE

A "Safe Cry Zone": Weathering the First Crisis

There's a newsletter about preventing child abuse that says, "Caring for your baby is not about stopping the crying. Caring for your baby is about *coping* with the crying."

As we have seen, crying can result in failed infant–parent relationships, the ultimate failure of which is child abuse. Now, to venture into some very dangerous and perhaps politically incorrect territory, here is another take on cultural differences, specifically shaken baby syndrome. We know that the number-one cause of shaken baby syndrome is crying and that most cases occur among people in poverty. Maybe shaken baby syndrome is not reported in the middle classes; maybe it does occur but we don't know about it. (This is the case with drug use; the poor are more likely to get reported for using illegal drugs.)

Maybe shaken baby syndrome is related to the learned helplessness of poverty. Maybe if you are living in a small apartment with paper-thin walls, the TV blaring, and five or six kids running around, a screaming baby or a baby crying all the time is just not thought of as unusual. It's just what babies do. Perhaps this subculture has redefined crying and taken the emergency part out. The siren has lost its power; it doesn't get anybody's attention until it's too late. By then the baby is so wound up that it would take massive efforts to calm him. The adult is so angry, impatient, and fed up that he is not going to be sensitive to the baby. You'll remember our sensitive, loving mom from chapter 4 who felt this way momentarily, and got help fast. Even if he knows how to calm the baby, at that moment he is incapable of anything but violence (most episodes of shaken baby syndrome are caused by the father or boyfriend).

Much is made of mothers who bring their babies to the emergency room (ER) because they can't handle their babies' crying. I say, good for them. They reached out and got help. Maybe it was help for the baby because the baby was really out of control and the mother couldn't calm him. Or maybe they were asking for help for themselves because they were afraid they would hurt their baby.

It's the parents who *don't* come to the ER that I worry about. We need to teach people to recognize crying as a problem before it is too late. If we change the perception that crying is "just what babies do" or that it is normal to hear a baby crying all the time, we can prevent abuse. We can prevent the baby from being shaken by not letting the episode escalate. Changing people's perceptions about crying would provide a tremendous public service. It would be difficult, but it is possible to change perceptions through education.

Shaken baby syndrome is such a horrific event. It is hard to imagine what it must feel like to reach the point where you would not only want to hurt a baby but actually do it. It suggests a total loss of control. The normal internal stops that prevent us from acting out our rage stop working.

When we fail to cope with crying, whether it's the extreme of shaken baby syndrome or something much less extreme, we stop seeing the baby as a baby. It reminds me of an optical illusion used in many psychology textbooks. It's a photo that is black on one side and white on the other. When you look at it you can either see a vase (the white side) or the profile of a face (the black side). But your brain won't let you see both at the same time. Maybe this is what happens with crying. We no longer see the baby in front of us. Our emotional brain, probably the limbic system, just can't handle the conflict, so we see something else, maybe an object of hate. At the very least, we stop seeing the baby as the helpless and innocent being we love.

Babies evoke intense feelings—both good and bad. It takes real anger and passion to even consider hurting a baby. But passion and anger mean you care. Dr. Brazelton likes to say,

"Value the passion." Once you recognize that negative emotions mean that you care, you can transform that energy into positive feelings or positive parenting to help the baby.

Yes, this is possible, though it may be hard to believe. Negative emotions can make us feel paralyzed. We become immobile. We feel like we can't do anything, or worse, that we will do something bad. And it's complicated. Being angry at your crying baby means that you have to deal with both the anger itself and what it means to you to be angry at your baby. You might be afraid that you are going to hurt the baby or, at the very least, not know what to do. If you can say to yourself, "I'm angry because I care, because I really want to help my baby, and I'm frustrated because I can't, and I feel helpless and inadequate," you will be freed from the prison of those negative feelings. When that happens, you can turn those negative feelings into positive feelings or at least positive action.

But what about when the passion is gone? Negative feelings at least mean that there are feelings to work with. When the passion is gone, the relationship is gone—or at the very least, it's a relationship in crisis. When the passion for parenting is gone, it can be replaced either by negative feelings or by emptiness. The baby no longer *is*. That is one thing that makes neglect different from abuse. Abuse is when you lose control over your intense feelings. Neglect is when you stop taking care of the baby because you just don't care anymore.

To manage a crying baby, you first have to understand that

you have the power to act. You then have to deal with the feelings inside. But finally, you need to develop an action plan. *You need to create a safe cry zone.*

Building a safe cry zone means practicing differentiated parenting. It also means knowing your "cryself," your internal warning signs and triggers. Go to your internal search engine and try to figure out your own reactions and feelings to your baby's crying. Examine how it makes you feel. What is it about the cry that bothers you—is it the amount, the sound? Are your feelings about how the crying is affecting your life? Your mate? Your marriage? Figure out what the triggers are for you. Where are the hot spots? When does it really get to you, and how do you feel when that happens?

Figure out the process of your internal buildup. Identify signs within yourself that you can recognize as your feelings build. If you can figure out your internal process, you will recognize the danger signs. What happens before you lose it? How do you know when you are headed in that direction? If you can forecast, you can short-circuit the process and prevent yourself from getting to a place that you don't want to be. You don't want to get trapped into a feeling state that immobilizes you. Learn to understand your internal pathways that lead to feeling imprisoned by your baby's crying. There are markers, signposts on the path. Find them and label them. Next time you see one, hang a left or a right. Pick up your internal clicker and change the channel.

The other advantage of doing this is that it gets easier the more you do it. If you understand how you feel about crying and what it is doing to you, you will be better able to cope. It won't be such a mystery. You won't be overcome by your feelings. You will recognize them when they come. It will be more like revisiting feelings you have had before. Maybe not pleasant feelings, but at least familiar. It takes the sting out. It's like saying to your feelings, "Hi there. I know you. I may not like you, but I've seen you before and I can deal with you."

Recognize and use your passion. As your anxiety or anger or immobility builds, say to yourself, "I'm really getting upset, but it means that I care and I love this baby, and I'm going to use these intense feelings to get myself mobilized and do something positive. I see the trap in the distance. I recognize I'm heading in that direction. So I hang a left and say, 'Baby, I really hate when you cry like this. I get so upset, I'm at my wits' end and feel like I can't do anything. But I know that I feel this way because of how much I care and knowing that makes me not afraid of these feelings. I can help you. So here, come to your dad!'" Becoming unstuck frees you up to take action, such as handing over the baby to someone else for a while. And that may be something that you've been unable to do before.

Once you have taken these three psychological steps—work on differentiated parenting, become familiar with your cryself, and use your passion—you will be well on your way to creating a safe cry zone. In this zone, your baby can cry, and you can respond calmly, without worry, anger, or guilt. You don't have to be perfect; just working on these steps will have beneficial effects. There's no test, no pop quiz, to help know when you're done. In fact, there's probably no such thing as being finished. This is an ongoing process. But just working on theses issues, thinking about them, and making them part of your parenting life will unburden you and make you better able to cope with crying. It will make you a better parent.

By now, you should feel that you can calm yourself down, that you have the tools, the skills, and the power, to do it. So steady yourself, take a step back, take stock of the situation, and decide what to do. And there are concrete things that can be done. When you feel less trapped by your baby's crying, you'll be more willing to try them. Here they are:

- *Get help with taking care of the baby.* Help can come in the form of a husband, a partner/significant other, a lover, or someone else, such as a friend, a family member, a neighbor, or an in-law. There are plenty of people out there who can take care of a crying baby. Hire a babysitter. The biggest reason parents say they won't leave the baby with anyone else is that they think the baby is too difficult to manage. "How can I leave her with a babysitter when she's going to cry the whole time?" How can you? You can because she is going to cry the whole time. You have to understand that you need and deserve a break. Getting a break from a screaming baby is not a luxury. It is not a sign of weakness. It does not mean that you are not up to the task of being a parent. It means that you are healthy and normal and have limits like any other human being. Give yourself credit for being normal. It means that you need your batteries recharged. It means that you can't be a good parent if you are depleted. You are doing both yourself and the baby a favor by letting other people help.

Frankly, if the baby is going to scream anyway, let her scream with somebody else! It's not like you're losing quality time. Give yourself a break, and then you will be getting quality time. I know you might feel bad about this, guilty leaving a crying baby with someone else. But it's not as if these feelings are going to go away. At least if you do something for yourself, you'll have something positive to counterbalance the guilt.

Of course, you owe it to babysitters or friends to warn them what they're in for and give them a chance to say no. But if they accept, take them at their word. Go out and have fun. Or at least go out. And don't take your cell phone.

I really do know how hard this is. In the Colic Clinic, we tell parents to go to a movie, have dinner, take a walk, anything. Just get away from the baby. But we don't just say it, because if we did, parents would always find excuses or say that they couldn't bring themselves to leave the baby with some else. Instead, we write the suggestion down, like a prescription. And it works. "My doctor said to do this," our parents say. "Look—it's right here. He wrote it down."

My hope is that after reading this book, you'll give yourself permission to leave your baby with someone else long enough to refresh yourself. Think of it as a prescription. In this culture, where we don't pick up each other's crying babies as a matter of course, parents need to know what resources are available and how to access them. If you think there may be times when you can't handle your baby's crying, set up a safety net ahead of time. Have someone close who has agreed to help you. Say, "Look, I may not need this, but if my baby is crying too much and I feel like I can't take it, will you take him for a while? Can I count on you?" Imagine how much better you would feel if you knew you had that kind of friend in the wings.

Mothers can get together and form support groups to spell each other when cry times are tough. Create a local network of helpers. There are other options as well. Find out if there are local hotlines or warmlines in your community to call for help. If not, get one started. Find out in advance if the ER is a realistic option, and if so, how to get there.

- *Get professional parenting help.* The hard part is giving yourself permission to get help, acknowledging that it is good for you and good for your baby. Many of the issues we deal with around colic are parenting stress issues. They can be handled by mental health professionals— psychologists, social workers, marriage and family counselors, and psychiatrists. Most insurance companies will reimburse for parenting distress. There is nothing wrong with you if get professional help for parenting. As I've said, I worry a lot more about the people who don't get help. Knowing that you need help is a huge step. It means you have recognized the problem. And asking for help means that you are willing to do something about it. These actions say good things about you, not bad things.

Getting help also means knowing what to do when the situation becomes critical, when you are in crisis. Keep phone numbers nearby of people you can call when you are desperate. An admirable group of single mothers set up a network of people they can call when they feel that they are over the top, desperate, and afraid that they might hurt their babies. These women know themselves well enough to know what they might do. They not only know their fears but also admit having them to others. What a great example of how the caring, the passion, behind the fear got turned into a protective net for the baby.

You can also help yourself by taking time out when your kid is screaming and you're alone and have no one to turn to. When you feel those warning signs coming on, put the baby in a safe place and take a shower. You can't hear the baby crying when you are in the shower, and no baby ever died from crying for 10 minutes. Put headphones on and listen to loud music. You can do this while you're carrying the baby. You're watching him. You can see what's going on. He's in your arms. He'll be fine. And it's a break for you.

Some mothers bring their babies to a hospital ER when they can't stop the crying and they have no other resources. Good for them. They know when they need help, and that is the first step.

There are also cry and colic support groups, parenting networks, and Internet chat rooms. One way to be proactive is to start your own cry support group. No matter where you are, you can't be too far from other families with infant cry problems.

You can also help yourself by keeping records. Using the Cry Diary (page 28) and the Colic Symptom Checklist (pages 29–34) we provided in chapter 2, you can keep track of your infant's crying to see if it is getting better or worse. This can be helpful too because it serves as a reality check. We've had parents say, "I felt like my baby's crying was getting worse, but I thought that I was imagining things. Then when I checked the records, I found out that she really was crying more. Then I knew I wasn't crazy!" We've also had mothers tell us the opposite. Some of these mothers were so exhausted that they felt like things were getting worse even when they weren't. These records can also be useful to bring to your pediatrician. He or she will probably appreciate that you did this and understand more about what you're going through. And the data might help with a referral or the development of a treatment plan.

- *Change the world.* There are things that we can do as a society to help with crying. We are not getting to people in time. We need to help people identify when crying is a problem sooner rather than later. We need to help them put a label on it while there is still time to get help. Before anyone blows. This means correctly identifying those infants with a cry problem and making sure they are not mislabeled as normal cryers. We need to help caregivers learn how to identify when the crying is becoming a problem for them early enough to get help. This kind of education can be done through parenting classes, obstetrical and pediatric visits, health clinics, as well as any media that reaches pregnant women and new mothers.

    Once people are better at identifying problem crying, we need to make sure they know what to do about it. This could mean community groups, self-help programs, and media presentations about coping strategies. Take-home packets that families get from hospitals could have this information. Visiting nurses could give it to mothers. The information could be made available wherever mothers go for obstetrical and pediatric checkups. Supermarkets and pharmacies are other good venues.

We need to enlist the health care system. Health care professionals need to ask about crying and not just assume that if the mother doesn't bring it up it's not on her mind or is not an issue. In fact, it could be a big issue, but she might be afraid to bring it up. She might be unwilling to say that she is afraid of hurting her baby when he cries. I understand that health care professionals have a lot to cover in a short time and that they have to set priorities. But I've always been struck, after many years of teaching pediatric residents, how often I've heard them say that the majority of questions they get at well-baby visits are in the area that they are least trained for and least comfortable with—behavior and development.

An article in a pediatric journal reported on a survey of maternal depression in mothers who brought their children in for well-baby checkups. The authors were alarmed at the high rate of maternal depression the study revealed, and they realized that no one was regularly identifying these mothers. The article suggested that screening for maternal depression should become a standard part of normal pediatrics visits. Great idea— especially given the double whammy that colic and depression represents.

This would be quite a departure from traditional pediatric care. And in the age of managed care, it's even more problematic. But there may be solutions. One is for health care professionals to have parents fill out a simple screening form while they sit in the waiting room. Then just before Mom gets called to see the doc, the nurse collects and quickly scores the form and gives it to the doctor along with the child's chart. The doc can then follow up if there are red flags for things such as crying or depression. Or Mom can complete the form at home and bring it in or mail it ahead of time.

Or we could change the health care reimbursement system so that screening for mental health and behavioral services could be reimbursed in the context of a medical visit. This would mean that the nurse's time for scoring the form and the doctor's time for reviewing it could be paid for. Another possibility would be to have behavioral and mental health services available at medical visits, either as part of the visit or in the same facility. This is one-stop shopping—and it's the model we use at the Colic Clinic. If pediatricians feel that screening for depression or dealing with things like crying are beyond the scope of what they want to do, let's have people there who can provide those services and let's make sure they're reimbursed.

If that happened, the pediatrician would become the gateway to other services in the one-stop shopping model. In the long run, it would probably be cheaper. And we'd save more lives and improve the quality of life for more families. We have to get it done somehow, because we're missing too many mothers and babies who need help.

What I've tried to offer you in this book is a way to deal with what is probably the first crisis in your relationship with your baby. Although you haven't even gotten past the first few months, what you've already learned about crying and parenthood should hold you in good stead throughout the parenting journey. How you resolve crying will shape how you deal with other bumps ahead in the parenting road. And crying will be back in other forms throughout your child's development, so you will get plenty of chances for instant replay. You will grow and learn and develop as parents, and as a family, and so will your infant. And crying will mean different things at different ages.

This is where education—or advance warning—is so helpful. By knowing why children cry at different ages, you can be better prepared. I'll tell you right now that crying increases with fear of strangers and the development of the attachment system toward the end of the first year. For example, the 14-month-old who loves the idea that she can now walk, will go into another room—only to discover that Mom is not there! She'll become terrified that you are gone forever and will scream. She'll also cry hard when you drop her off at day care.

You know you're coming back, but she doesn't. You need to know in advance that the toddler temper tantrum is not about you. It's about the baby. It's about her frustration. And then there's the first day of school. Can she let go? Can you?

But as important as education is, don't kid yourself into thinking that the answers are all "out there" rather than within yourself. There is no denying that we live in a society that has seen the breakdown of the nuclear family, where fewer people have the experience of growing up in large extended families and learn to take care of babies. So we approach parenthood feeling somewhat clueless about parenting and what babies are all about. We feel incompetent to parent and at the same experience a sense of social isolation because there is little family around. And we feel this way in an age of information explosion, when there are more books and Web sites and experts on parenting than we can keep track of. This makes us feel even more inadequate. These feelings are real and part of our society, part of our culture. You need to balance these feelings with the knowledge and an inner confidence that you already know how to parent. There are plenty of answers within you. Human beings were born to parent. So much of parenting is intuitive. Go ahead and click and double-click—but also look within yourself.

Understanding that many of the things we Americans do as parents are because our culture has developed that way helps take the right and wrong out of parenting. We no longer have to say, "It's okay for babies to cry all day." We can recognize the legitimacy of feeling that it is not okay for babies to cry a lot, and can stop the feeling that we have to either let the crying continue or end it with anger and violence. Let's start a new culture—a culture with a safe cry zone where we understand what our babies are trying to tell us.

Crying in early infancy is the first of so many more tests to come. You never have to be a victim of your child's crying. So start early. There's so much at stake. Make parenting happen the way you want it to. Use your passion. Value yourself. I know you can do it.

INDEX

Page numbers in italics refer to figures.

Index

Index

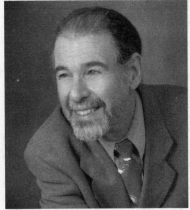

PHOTO CREDIT: RCL Portrait Design

Barry M. Lester, Ph.D. is director of the Infant Development Center at Women & Infants Hospital in Providence, Rhode Island, which houses the Colic Clinic. He is also professor of psychiatry and human behavior and professor of pediatrics at Brown Medical School.

Catherine O'Neill Grace is the coauthor with Michael Thompson, Ph.D., and Lawrence J. Cohen, Ph.D., of *Best Friends, Worst Enemies: Understanding the Social Lives of Children* and *Mom, They're Teasing Me: Helping Your Child Solve Social Problems*. She has also written many nonfiction books for children, among them *The White House: An Illustrated History* (Scholastic, 2003). She lives in Buffalo, New York.